NURTURING
SUPERWOMAN

THE BUSY WOMAN'S GUIDE TO
STRESS REDUCTION AND DYNAMIC HEALTH

*Hormone harmony is the secret to women's health,
while stress and doing too much lead to hormone chaos.
Start nurturing your hormones and create dynamic health!*

To Miriam
best wishes
Carolyn Moody
14/4/03

NURTURING SUPERWOMAN
THE BUSY WOMAN'S GUIDE TO
STRESS REDUCTION AND DYNAMIC HEALTH

First published in 2003 by Abacus Communications
Avenue de l'Europe 45 - 1330 Rixensart - Belgium

Cover design and layout by Studio Dewit
Brusselsesteenweg 593 - 3090 Overijse - Belgium

Printing and binding by Printing Poot
Industrielaan 12 - 1702 Groot-Bijgaarden - Belgium

ISBN 2-9600345-0-3

This book has been printed on chlorine-free paper.

Disclaimers

The information contained within this document has been carefully checked and is believed to be entirely reliable and consistent with the issues that it describes. However, no responsibility is assumed for inaccuracies nor does Personal Health Development, Carolyn Moody, Dip I.O.N., Optimum Nutrition & Lifestyle Therapist, Belgium & UK assume any liability arising out of the issues described herein.

The information contained in this book is for information purposes only. It should not be used as a substitute for professional medical diagnosis and care. Do not attempt to self diagnose and do seek medical advice about any symptoms before embarking on a nutrition programme.

CONTENTS

Dedication

I have dedicated this book to Gemma, my beautiful daughter. She represents the next generation of bright young women who seek truth and enlightenment in a world where self interest and the bottom line count for more than the pursuit of excellent health.

Acknowledgements

I owe my thanks to a great many people who have helped me to make this book a reality. It was a long time in the making but so many people have encouraged me, persuaded me that I could do it, and helped in so many practical ways.

Paul for being a constant in my life and for rescuing me from many frustrating computer problems.

Kathy, Dave, Bettina and Heather for volunteering to proofread just when I despaired of ever being able to see and correct all my own mistakes.

Steve and Marianne for their belief in me, their constant encouragement and all their ideas and suggestions.

Steve and Pauline for running the first book shop and natural health centre to say they wanted to promote and sell my book.

Babara S for so much practical input, helping me make my nutrition consultancy and my book a success.

Barbara P for telling me I should write a book - long before I had even thought of it.

Doreen for showing me that all of my established written material was in fact embrionic books just waiting to be developed.

Hugo for designing a beautiful cover and for his endless patience.

All my friends and family for taking such an interest and spurring me on to complete this first book and having enough faith to say they will buy a copy for themselves and their friends, before they'd even seen it.

CAROLYN MOODY, Dip I.O.N., and PERSONAL HEALTH DEVELOPMENT

"There is more to health than just eating the right food. Equally as important are having a healthy relationship with food (not using it to deal with emotional issues) and a balanced lifestyle that includes adequate relaxation, rest, sleep, exercise, connected relationships and fulfilling work."
Carolyn Moody

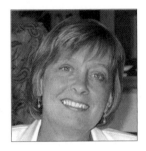

Carolyn trained as a Nutritional Therapist at the Institute for Optimum Nutrition (I.O.N.) in London, qualifying in 1990. Founded in the early 1980s by Patrick Holford, I.O.N. is a well known and respected organisation in the UK, with an unsurpassed reputation for the high standard of its training courses.

Since 1990, under the title of Personal Health Development, Carolyn has been helping people make more balanced nutritional and lifestyle choices in Belgium, the UK and Jersey through her workshops, presentations, consultations and published work.

Many of Carolyn's clients are referred to her by their doctors for a wide variety of health problems, including women's health issues, unresolvable digestive problems, raised cholesterol, blood sugar and blood pressure, chronic fatigue and weight. The rest of her client work is through personal recommendation. With the growth in popularity of email, Carolyn now has a fast expanding business in 'distance consultations' via email and 'phone.

As well as being an experienced educator, Carolyn is a respected writer on nutrition issues, having many published articles, including the I.O.N. Journal and a regular column for an aviation magazine on 'human factors', covering such topics as pilot fatigue and error, cosmic radiation and the effect of jet lag. This is the first of a planned series of books by Carolyn on various aspects of nutrition and health.

FORWARD

by Dr. D. Van der Mijnsbrugge, M.D.

I started working in Brussels as a General Practitioner in 1980. Disillusioned with the limitations of the mainstream medical approach to health problems and having always been interested in the effects of nutrition on health, I studied with the Ortho Institute in the Netherlands, qualifying in 1989.

The Ortho Institute is a Dutch foundation that provides information and training on nutrition and health. Its philosophy is based on that defined by two times Nobel Prize Laureate, Linus Pauling (Science 1968; 160:265-271). The Institute's president, Gert Schuitemaker, is also president of the International Society for Orthomolecular Medicine (ISOM) based in Toronto, Canada.

Many of my patients with hormonal problems have responded well to the nutritional approach. However, being a busy GP means I don't usually have sufficient time to discuss in detail diet, supplements and how to incorporate the recommended changes. To have more background information about the causes of hormonal imbalance and disturbance, I welcome "*Nurturing Superwoman.*" This book is vital reading for every woman who wants to know more about how her hormones work and the nutritional influences on their health. It is also an important reference for doctors who are interested in the nutritional approach to hormone health. Succinct enough that busy women do not have to spend too much time trying to retrieve appropriate information, the book contains sufficient detail to answer most patients' questions.

I am impressed with the research that has gone into this book, and with the clearly laid out format of the material. The nutritional information is particularly valuable, especially the addition of meal planners, recipes and practical advice on how to shop and prepare healthy meals. I hope to see this book translated into both Dutch and French, as I think the Dutch and French speaking communities in Belgium, Holland and France would appreciate the information it contains.

My congratulations to Carolyn Moody for an excellent nutrition guide to women's hormone health, and I look forward to seeing the next in her series of planned books.

INTRODUCTION

Women in the 21st century are still suffering from the legacy of the 70s Superwoman who thought she could have it all - career, home, family, relationships, social life, independence – and that it should all be done perfectly. This has become such an entrenched part of the female psyche that women don't realise they are doing too much and letting good nutritional habits slide. The result is too much stress, leading to fatigue as well as digestive and hormone-related health problems.

Despite the plethora of health books aimed at women, there is still much confusion around hormones. Many women are just not aware they have hormones until something goes wrong with their health. When the doctor diagnosed hormone imbalance in my friend's 21 year old daughter, my friend (now entering the menopause) said to me:

"But how can that be? Young women don't have hormone problems. Hormones only affect women going into the menopause, don't they?"

From puberty until the menopause, a women's hormones have an enormous impact on her overall health, vitality, mental stability and wellbeing. Get the balance right and life is sweet music. Out of balance and life can be hell. One of the most frightening things any woman can hear is the diagnosis of breast, uterine, ovarian or cervical cancer, all of which are related to hormone health. I hope the information contained in this book will help women understand their hormone health better and find ways of maintaining balance and harmony to avoid developing serious disease.

Too much to do

While there are many environmental and nutritional influences on hormone problems, I believe an important factor is the stress created by women trying to do too much. Many of the women I see are trying to work long hours, run a home, bring up children, have a social life, and be a wonderful partner. Something has to give – usually good eating habits. Because of so many pressures, women have less time and energy for meal planning, shopping and cooking. They tend to eat whatever is convenient and to hand, and to keep going with cups of coffee, sugary snacks and regular alcohol consumption. There is very little time to fit in regular exercise or for rest, relaxation and sufficient sleep. With exhaustion and less than adequate nutrition, comes less resistance to hormonal imbalances.

Once they start going through the menopause, women can often feel a loss of confidence (sometimes experienced as sheer panic!) as their bodies undergo changes that can leave them feeling out of control. Assertive women, used to organising families, high powered jobs and a hectic social life, may suddenly feel as though they are going mad. They lose concentration, can't remember things, can't seem to get a decent, unbroken night's sleep any more, suffer lack of energy and feel more tired than usual. And all of this on top of hot flushes, night sweats, loss of sex drive, painful intercourse, weight gain, aching joints, lowered immunity, and developing allergies out of the blue.

The menopause can be just one more stress for women who are already expending a lot of energy juggling too many balls in the air. It is a time of immense change in a woman's life: an emotional time and the end of an era when she says goodbye to her fertile years – and her youth. The good news is that many women come into their own after they have stopped having periods and they are no longer governed by the monthly ups and downs of oestrogen and progesterone. Testosterone levels may rise slightly giving them what has been described as 'postmenopausal zest'. Energy levels rise and women find they feel more assertive, independent of other people's approval and healthier than they did when they were younger. Many women change careers or channel all their new found energy into doing something they always wanted to do, but never had time for during their menstruating and childbearing years.

Maintaining balance

The secret to a healthy menopause is the same as for the menstruating years. Keeping hormones in harmony through balanced nutrition and a healthy lifestyle is the natural way for women to live. Optimum nutrition is a holistic approach that encourages women to take back responsibility for their health. Depending on the severity of the imbalances, optimum nutrition works well on its own, or in combination with orthodox treatments.

Women's health problems respond particularly well to the nutritional approach to healing. In all the years I have been practising I have never failed to be amazed, and delighted, at the results of a well balanced nutrition programme in helping people regain their sense of wellbeing and good health.

Irene's story

One of the very first women I ever saw in consultation, Irene, came to see me because her periods had stopped and she had started growing hair on the back of her hands and on her face (hirsuitism). Irene's doctor confirmed with a blood test that she was producing virtually no oestrogen and her testosterone levels had gone sky high. The solution was to take the Pill, which did indeed return her hormone levels to normal and give her back her periods. Unfortunately, Irene put on a lot of weight and felt very depressed taking the Pill and stopped after a couple of months. This caused the original hormonal imbalance to resurface with all the accompanying symptoms of hirsuitism.

Irene, who was a vibrant and attractive women in her mid-thirties, was feeling a bit desperate by the time I saw her. I recommended a diet and supplement programme that included Vitex Agnus Castus, telling her that it was my first experience using this herb. We were both delighted when three months later her periods were back to normal and her doctor confirmed with a blood test that her hormone profile was well within the normal range. Irene's hair growth had also returned to normal. This was the first of many confirmations that the natural solutions to women's health problems are very effective, whether it is treating PMS, menopausal symptoms, flooding periods, lack of periods or endometriosis.

About this book

This is the first in a series of nutrition guides that has grown out of my contact with many people thirsting for the knowledge that will help them achieve and maintain their potential for excellent health. The majority of them are women. While these days men do take more interest in their health, it's a sad fact that most still rely on their women folk to take care of them. It is therefore fitting that the first in my series of nutrition guides is dedicated to women's health.

Despite being told by a number of publishing houses that the market is "*already saturated*" with books about nutrition and women's health, I have received a great deal of support and many requests for this book to be written from the many women with whom I come into contact. Men have also told me they would like a copy for their partners – as well as to increase their own knowledge and understanding. This is what decided me to go ahead and self-publish. The women for whom I have written this book usually don't have the time or energy to go hunting for the appropriate title in their local book store. They want access to good information, written in an easy to read style, that can be picked up and delved into when they have the odd moment.

More than a "what to eat" book

"Nurturing Superwoman" isn't just another 'what to eat' book – there are plenty of those around already. My experience shows that women want to know the 'why' - *"why will changing my diet and taking supplements make any difference to my PMS...?"* and the 'how', as in *"how do I apply all this knowledge?"* With this in mind I have included useful background information on how women's hormones work, the environmental and nutritional influences on hormonal health, and some natural solutions based on diet, vitamin, mineral, essential fatty acid supplements, and herbal and plant remedies that have stood the test of time.

Most important is a seven day meal planner with a shopping list and recipes to get you started with practical ideas on applying the recommendations.

The information in this book will help you achieve hormone harmony right the way through from puberty to 60 plus. It is based on current knowledge of the effects of food, supplements, herbs and lifestyle on a woman's endocrine system, but new research is throwing up more information almost on a daily basis. I have credited the many wonderful authors who have inspired me and included a reference list of just a fraction of the many studies that have taken place in the last thirty or forty years.

All the women with whom I have come into contact have taken such an intelligent and searching interest in their health, that what I hope I have finally achieved is to answer the questions that they have asked me. This book grew out of that objective.

Working with a doctor

I now work in both the UK and Belgium, with my main practice still in Belgium. I was fortunate enough when I first qualified to come across a doctor who was trained in orthomolecular medicine (nutritional medicine). Dr Van der mijnsbrugge, who wrote the forward to this book, has been a great help to me and my clients when they have needed medical diagnosis and diagnostic testing. He has also been able to provide more intensive treatment, such as intravenous vitamin and mineral therapy, for those with severe health problems who need a more drastic approach to balancing the imbalances.

A number of doctors also refer their patients to me, particularly those who have requested a different approach to their health problems other than long term medication, or those who can no longer tolerate hormone medication.

Case histories

Because I know that people like to hear about other's experiences, I have used examples of case histories throughout this book, based on women I have met over the years as well as my own experiences. In order to protect identity, all names have been changed.

Not a substitute for medical diagnosis and care

Please use this book to help you become informed about the natural choices you can make for your health. Do not use it as a substitute for professional medical diagnosis and care. It is important that you do not attempt to self diagnose and that you seek medical advice about any of your symptoms before embarking on a nutrition programme. Before I see anyone for a consultation, I ask them to have a thorough check up with their medical practitioner. I then prefer there to be a cooperative interaction between myself, the client and her supervising doctor, with the client's best interests always the focus of attention.

Finally, like many women before you, I hope you too will gain some insights into your hormonal problems in the pages of this book, and I wish you the best of health !

Carolyn Moody, Dip I.O.N.,
Optimum Nutrition & Lifestyle Therapist

PART ONE

HOW HORMONES AFFECT HEALTH, MENTAL STABILITY AND WELLBEING

CHAPTER 1
CHAOS VERSUS HARMONY

Chaos and disharmony

Premenstrual syndrome, fibroids, cysts, heavy, painful and irregular periods, endometriosis, polycystic ovaries, infertility, menopause, hot flushes, osteoporosis, loss of sex drive, lack of energy, depression, irritability, breast, uterine and cervical cancer ...

It reads like a catalogue of misery designed to make women's lives as unbearable as possible! But these are just symptoms that show how women's health is being subject to environmental and nutritional influences on an unprecedented scale. All of the above are related to the health and balance of your hormones.

How can your hormones be so involved in all of the above health problems, and what can you do for yourself to achieve and maintain hormone balance and health?

Balance and harmony

A woman's hormones have a big impact on both her physical and emotional well-being – as any woman caught up in the monthly emotional see-saw of PMS will tell you. Female hormones are designed to work in perfect harmony, much like a well conducted orchestra. When your hormones are in proper balance you feel emotionally and physically well. Life is great music. Nature has even designed the menopause as a gradual decline in hormone levels over a number of years to avoid just the kind of upheaval that so many women experience. With good nutrition and a healthy lifestyle your hormones should stay in harmony and the transition from menstruation to menopause should be relatively smooth, with minimum side effects.

With your hormones in balance, the probability of developing hormone related conditions such as breast, ovarian and uterine cancer diminishes, as does the incidence of endometriosis, fibroids, cysts, osteoporosis and infertility. No matter what your genetic predisposition, e.g. having close relatives who have developed breast cancer, it is not inevitable that you will suffer from the same health problems. It just means that you may need to be more conscious of the importance of maintaining healthy genes and a strong immune system.

First Indications of hormone distress

It is when your hormones stop working in harmony that you feel out of balance and start experiencing hormone distress. In the menstruating years, this can take the form of premenstrual syndrome (PMS), while during the menopausal years, you may experience a number of unpleasant symptoms.

The following list gives you an idea of all the symptoms and conditions that are usually related to hormonal dis-ease or dis-stress.

- **Premenstrual syndrome**: fatigue, depression, irritability, mood swings, tender breasts, abdominal cramping, backache, headaches, insomnia
- **Period problems**: severe heavy bleeding (menorrhagia), painful periods (dysmenorrhoea), irregular periods, cessation or absence of periods (amenorrhoea)
- **Lumps and growths (benign)**: fibroids, cysts, polycystic ovaries
- **Endometriosis**
- **Cancer**: breast, uterine, ovarian and cervical cancer
- **Infertility**
- **Menopause**: hot flushes, night sweats, emotional outbursts, depression, anxiety, loss of sex drive, vaginal dryness and pain during intercourse, loss of concentration and memory, lack of energy, allergies, lowered immunity, joint pain
- **Osteoporosis** and loss of bone density

Stress – the cause of hormone dysfunction ?

The fundamental cause of all of the above symptoms is stress, hence hormonal dis-stress. This causes some confusion as stress is normally associated with the feelings generated around being stuck in a traffic jam, suffering a bereavement, having an argument with the boss or spouse, moving house – in effect any form of emotional stress. However, there are four different kinds of stress, all of which represent a challenge to your health on a daily basis. The four sources of stress are :

(1) **Emotional** (includes both current and unresolved chronic emotional stress), e.g. worries about job, money, relationship, children, a loss or bereavement, moving house, living in a culture not your own, overwork, being bored at work, unresolved relationship problems with family members ...

(2) **Physical**, e.g. too much or too little exercise, pain, infection, ill health, fatigue, unsuitable working environment, prescription or recreational drugs, synthetic hormones (i.e. the Pill or HRT), pregnancy, dental fillings (both amalgam and

14

composite), tobacco smoke, cigarettes, autotoxicity, leaky gut, candidiasis …

(3) **Environmental**, e.g. pollution found in pesticides, herbicides and nitrates from artificial fertilizers on food and in water, dioxins and other industrial pollution, tyre wear, car exhaust, environmental oestrogens …

(4) **Nutritional**, e.g. caffeine, sugar, refined foods, high acidic diet, alcohol, junk food, processed fats, microwave dinners, fizzy drinks, rushing meals, eating on the run, eating too fast, not chewing food, allergies and food intolerance, eating too few vegetables and fruit, nutritional deficiencies, unbalanced vegetarian diet, very low calorie weight loss programmes, latest fad diets…

When your hormones get out of balance it is usually due to a culmination of a number of different stressors that may have been building up over a period of time.

Homeostasis – the drive for equilibrium

I have always thought that what is more amazing than the fact that people get sick because of the bombardment of stress in 21st century life, is the fact that so many people seem to survive, and even thrive. It's a testament to the body's incredible ability to maintain homeostasis (relatively stable equilibrium). It can be very encouraging to know that, no matter how bad or unwell you feel, your body is expending an enormous amount of energy trying to achieve and maintain good health. Even if you feel as though you are falling apart mentally and physically due to hormone chaos, just keep reminding yourself that your body isn't deliberately trying to make your life a misery. Quite the opposite, your symptoms are a sign that all is not well but if you provide the conditions needed for healing, your body will do its very best to get well.

Clearing away the debris

Some forms of stress you can do nothing about, such as the levels of pollution in the world or your working environment, but removing as many as you can will be like lifting a burden off the body's homeostatic mechanism. For those who have ever taken over a completely wild and overgrown garden, you will know that in order to return the garden to beauty, productivity and a haven for wildlife, you have to clear away all the choking weeds, dead and diseased plants, and then replenish the soil with valuable nutrients and live compost. Plants grown in optimum conditions grow strong and lush. If conditions are not ideal, the same plants will be weak and prey to attack by pests. In ideal conditions, your hormones will stay

15

balanced and you will feel well. All your stressors are like the overgrowth choking the life out of the garden. Remove as many of these as possible and your health will flourish. Take Janet as an example.

Janet's story

Janet sought help because of severe PMS one week before each period. Other symptoms included exhaustion, digestive problems, abdominal bloating, pain and wind, constipation, cravings for sweet things, lack of sex drive, headaches, weight gain, heavy periods and pain, joint and muscle aches and pains, hayfever, sinusitis, insomnia, feelings of anxiety, tension and irritability, and frequent colds and chest infections.

Working full time and trying to bring up two small children, Janet led a very stressful life. Each morning she was up at 6 a.m. and on the road by 7 a.m. to take the children to a crèche before trying to beat the traffic and get to work at 8 a.m. Each evening she did the reverse journey, sitting in heavy traffic for an hour, arriving home around 7 p.m. She then fed her children and got them to bed and started preparing a meal for when her husband arrived home at 8.30 p.m. They rarely sat down to eat before 9 p.m.

Janet was so hungry when she got home from work that she usually finished up whatever the children left on their plates and snacked on cheese and biscuits while she was preparing the evening meal. She wasn't really hungry by 9 p.m., but it was the only time she and her husband had together, and they usually relaxed by sharing a bottle of wine between them. Janet would fall into bed around midnight and then sleep badly. Her children were often awake in the night which also disturbed her sleep.

Janet's job was very busy which left her little time to take a break from her desk. When I checked her eating habits I found Janet was skipping breakfast (no time and it was too early in the morning to eat) and grabbing a croissant and coffee in the canteen. She drank about 4 cups of strong black coffee a day, 2 cups of black tea, and had one or two diet cokes from the machine near her office. About mid-afternoon she regularly had a chocolate bar with her tea or coffee because she was so exhausted and needed the stimulation to keep going.

Lunch was a cheese or ham sandwich and the evening meal was usually something quick based around pasta, meat and usually some salad, but not always.

When I added up all Janet's daily stressors they made quite a list :

- Bringing up a very young family
- Working long hours
- A lot of time on the road between work, crèche and home
- No exercise
- Too much time spent indoors in artificial lighting and recycled air
- Hours of exposure to electromagnetic fields (computer, fax machine, photocopier)
- Not enough fresh air or sunshine
- Sleep deprivation leading to extreme fatigue
- Overuse of stimulants, such as tea, coffee, alcohol, chocolate and cola drinks
- Insufficient fruit and vegetables and too much reliance on convenience foods based on wheat and dairy produce
- Nutritional deficiencies right across the board due to poor diet and loss of nutrients caused by too many stimulants and chronic stress
- Eating late in the evening and going to bed on a full stomach
- Poor digestion and absorption due to low levels of stomach acid and digestive enzymes
- Poor elimination caused by disrupted intestinal flora and lack of fibre
- No time for rest, relaxation or self

There was a lot to deal with here, but over time Janet reorganised her life, working part time closer to home. She changed her dietary habits to include more fresh food and relied a lot less on processed food and nutritional stressors to keep her going. She also stopped drinking during the week and just had between 2 and 4 glasses of wine at weekends. Not only did she lose weight easily, but she also started sleeping better and had more energy during the day. All her other symptoms gradually disappeared over the next three to four months. In the end, nutritional support was only part of the solution for Janet. She also had to make some pretty radical lifestyle changes in order to sustain her recovery and regain her hormone balance.

CHAPTER 2
ENVIRONMENTAL STRESS

Environmental stress is one of the stressors that you cannot avoid completely. It comes in many forms. Pollution from pesticides, nitrates, industrial fallout like dioxins, lead and cadmium, car emissions, tyre wear and cigarette smoke affects our food, water and the air we breathe. We are constantly exposed to chemical pollution from fungicides and the chemicals present in the synthetic materials used in our homes, work places and all public buildings. Environmental stress also includes the noise from city life, electromagnetic forces from our TV sets, computers and other electrical equipment so vital to 21st century living, and from microwaves emitted by microwave ovens and mobile phones. All this adds up to a lot of environmental stress. No wonder our health is suffering!

Oestrogen dominance

In his book, *"Hormonal Sabotage"*, Dr. Theo Colban describes a form of pollution that is causing particular concern among the scientific establishment. Oestrogen dominance is having a huge impact on our hormonal health, including that of animal life on land and in rivers and seas.[1] *"We are drowning in a sea of oestrogens"*, said David Feldman, Stanford University. These xenoestrogens (xeno meaning strange or foreign) come from petrochemical derivatives, including pesticides, herbicides and plastics, and hormones such as HRT and the Pill. They all have a phenol ring in common with our own oestrogen as part of their molecular structure and are able to mimic our oestrogens, fooling the body into accepting them in place of those produced by the body. It is feared they are wreaking havoc on human and animal fertility.[2]

According to Frank Comhaire, Professor of Endocrinology at Gent University, pesticide levels in Flanders, Belgium, are five times higher than in the Netherlands or Germany. Pesticides are one of the main sources of oestrogen mimics on our food.[3] A European Commission study confirms Professor Comhaire's claims. It found that pesticide residues in 7.4 per cent of Belgian fruit and vegetable samples exceeded the MRLs (Maximum Residue Levels) permitted by national and EU laws. By contrast, the average for the 15 EU member countries, plus Norway, Iceland and Finland was only 4.3 per cent. Lettuce and lemons contained the highest residue levels, while cauliflower was found to contain no traces of dangerous substances. In a UK government report from the Pesticides Residues Committee of 1999, 43 percent of fresh fruit and vegetables revealed the presence of pesticide residues – up from 33 per cent the year before.[4]

None of the other steroid hormones, such as testosterone, progesterone or corticosterone, share this same phenol ring structure, which is why scientists are so concerned about the rise of oestrogen in the environment. Oestrogen dominance implies a lowering of progesterone levels and it is this imbalance in menstruating women that can lead to so many hormone-related problems. In postmenopausal women there is a natural halt to the output of progesterone from the ovaries creating a state of unopposed oestrogen. Normally postmenopausal women should produce sufficient progesterone and oestrogen in the adrenals to balance each other. If there are too many environmental oestrogens upsetting this delicate balance, and the adrenals are not able to produce enough natural progesterone, then oestrogen dominance can occur. This in turn can lead to cancer and osteoporosis, as well as a whole host of health problems.

Environmental oestrogens and hormone-related cancers

First signs of oestrogen dominance were noticed among wildlife, particularly alligators in the Everglades in Florida. However, human beings are affected too. Between 1938 and 1990, sperm count among men dropped about 50% and the quality of sperm was affected. On top of this the rate of testicular cancer has tripled and that of prostate cancer has doubled.

The increase in oestrogens is lowering levels of progesterone, and is being blamed for the rise in breast and uterine cancer in women in the last twenty years. Oestrogen dominance is the only known cause of uterine cancer. Twenty years ago, 1 in 20 women could expect to get breast cancer in Europe and the US. Now it's around 1 in 10, with the highest risk group being women over the age of forty. The World Health Organisation estimates that each year more than 1.2 million people will be diagnosed with breast cancer worldwide.[6,7]

PCBs, dioxin and endometriosis

PCBs (polychlorinated biphenyls) and dioxin are both forms of environmental pollution. They are xenoestrogens in that they have a molecular structure similar to our own oestrogens. PCBs are used in plastics for food packaging and dioxin is involved in the bleaching industry. Women exposed to PCBs and dioxin have higher rates of breast cancer and some research has revealed that women with endometriosis have high levels of PCBs and dioxin in their blood.[8,9]

Endometriosis is a condition where the lining of the uterus grows outside the uterus, usually in the abdominal cavity, for example attached to intestines. When the uterus lining is shed and bleeds once a month, so does the endometrial tissue – wherever it has transplanted itself. PCBs and dioxin both interfere with the immune system as well as the endocrine system, and it is this disruption that is believed to cause endometriosis. But they are not the only culprits. Dr. Colborn has shown that at least 45 chemicals widely distributed in the environment, including 35 pesticides and 10 industrial chemicals, can damage the endocrine and immune systems. No doubt there are many more chemicals which have a disastrous effect on our health.

Hormones in water and food packaging

To add to this rise in environmental oestrogens, women are prescribed synthetic oestrogens in the form of the Pill or HRT to treat a number of hormonal problems. Not only are these synthetic hormones adding to the oestrogen dominance in the body of the woman taking them, but they are also getting back into the water cycle – flushed down the toilet and back into our rivers and the sea. So everyone, men, women and children are consuming hormones in drinking water – whether they want them or not.

To avoid the danger from food packaging, it is important to avoid butter and margarine in plastic tubs, metal cans lined with plastic, greenhouse vegetables that are sprayed with high levels of pesticides, plastic containers used to store food in the fridge, baby bottles, mineral water bottles and garden chemicals. Xenoestrogens are stored in fat, whether it is our own or in animal fat, butter, margarine, cheese, milk and anything made with them. Vegetarians may do slightly better than meat eaters because they avoid the fat that is an integral part of even the leanest muscle meat. However, unless they are buying organic vegetables and avoiding milk products, they too will be exposed to a wide range of xenoestrogens.

It's not just food packaging that contains these oestrogen mimics. Household detergents break down to release xenoestrogens, and dioxin (used in bleaching paper and as fallout from city incinerators) is a potent oestrogen mimic. Ways to avoid environmental oestrogens are :

• Avoid plastic packaging on your food as much as possible
• Eat only organic food where available
• Say 'no' to hormone medication unless absolutely necessary and then ask your doctor for natural oestrogen and progesterone.
• Use vinegar-based cleaning products
• Buy only non-bleached paper
• Avoid tampons and sanitary towels that have been bleached with dioxin
• Garden organically if you can, avoiding the use of pesticides and herbicides

Symptoms associated with oestrogen dominance

When the delicate balance between oestrogens and progesterone is disturbed, and particularly when oestrogens dominate at the expense of progesterone, women will suffer from a variety of symptoms.[10]

- Anovulatory menstrual cycles (i.e. no ovulation)
- PMS
- Weight gain
- Menstrual cycle irregularity
- Infertility
- Menopausal symptoms
- Osteoporosis
- Endometriosis
- Fibroids
- Fibrocystic breast disease
- Uterine and breast cancer
- Abnormal thyroid function

The cause of oestrogen dominance is due to a variety of factors, one of them being the influence of environmental oestrogens, but also the effect of poor nutrition, nutritional deficiencies and stress.

Nature's answer - phytoestrogens

Phyto (meaning plant) estrogens are natural components of plant foods. They have a similar structure to human oestrogens and are able to act as an anti-oestrogenic agent by locking on to the body's oestrogen receptor sites, thereby blocking the effect of both environmental oestrogens and an excess of 'home-produced' oestrogens. Through their weak oestrogenic activity, phytoestrogens are thought to rebalance a woman's own hormones, raising levels that are too low and lowering them when they are too high. They may well be helpful in reducing the risk of breast cancer by suppressing or inhibiting normal oestrogenic activity in breast tissue.[11]

According to Dr. Barbour Warren, Ph.D, Research Associate at Cornell University,[12] more than 300 foods have been shown to contain phytoestrogens. They are found in the seeds, stems, roots or flowers of plants, where they serve as natural fungicides that act as part of the plant's defence mechanism against micro organisms. All foods of plant origin, e.g. fruit, vegetables (including potatoes), pulses, seeds, nuts, wholegrains, spices and seaweed contain phytoestrogens. Eggs also contain phytoestrogens.

There are three main types of phytoestrogens: isoflavones, coumestans and lignans. Isoflavones are particularly abundant in pulses (legumes), especially soya beans and fermented soya products. The consumption of fermented soya, such as tofu, miso and tempeh in the traditional diet of Asian women is believed to be the reason for their low incidence of breast cancer.

Coumestan, found in various beans such as split peas, pinto beans and lima beans, alfalfa and red clover (the latter two having the highest amounts of coumestan), is less well researched but has been found to have strong interactions with oestrogen receptors in the body and therefore oestrogen-like activity. In fact red clover is used commercially either in a herbal preparation, or in conjunction with wild yam cream, to help regulate women's hormonal imbalances.

Lignans (a form of fibre) are an important source of phytoestrogens for Western women as they are found in all fibre-rich foods, including whole grains, (e.g. wheat, oats, rye, barley and rice), beans and linseeds. The phytoestrogenic quality of linseed is also found in the oil and flour made from the seeds.

Studies show that women with breast cancer have lower levels of lignan phytoestrogens in their urine than women without cancer, suggesting that it is important to eat plenty of fibre and phytoestrogen-rich fruit, vegetables, nuts, seeds and pulses on a regular basis.[13]

CHAPTER 3
HORMONE CASCADE

Hormones are chemical messengers secreted by a specific gland in the endocrine system into the blood where they travel to an appropriate cell to carry out their function. Once a hormone reaches its target cell, it attaches to a receptor site, like a key fitting a lock. When the receptor site is full it is unable to accept another load. Hormones work on a feedback system - when oestrogen is dominant in the first half of the menstrual cycle, it blocks the receptor sites in the uterus for progesterone, and vice versa in the second half of the cycle.[14] This system is upset when synthetic hormones enter the body and take up receptor sites in breast and uterine tissue, blocking their availability to the body's own hormones. Diagram 1 shows the different parts of the female endocrine system.

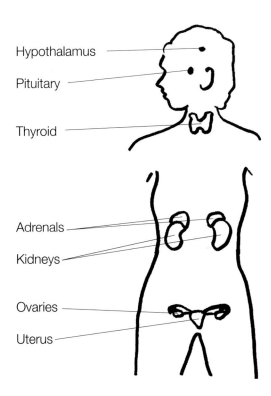

Hypothalamus

Pituitary

Thyroid

Adrenals

Kidneys

Ovaries

Uterus

Diagram 1. Female endocrine system

The female menstrual cycle is orchestrated by a number of different hormones, conducted by the hypothalamus. The hypothalamus weighs less than 28 gms of grey matter in the brain, yet is responsible for behaviour, emotional responses and for balancing everything that goes on automatically in the body. This includes the body's temperature, rate of metabolism and sleep, growth, hunger, thirst, blood chemistry and respiration. It does this by passing hormonal messages on to other parts of the endocrine system, including the pituitary gland, thyroid, ovaries and adrenal glands. The pituitary and the ovaries are the most closely linked to the production of oestrogens and progesterone during the menstruating years, with the pituitary acting as the conductor and maintaining a balance among the different hormones.[15] However, because of the connection between all parts of the endocrine system, if the thyroid or adrenals are thrown out of balance, it can effect the overall balance of hormones.

The influence of the hypothalamus on the rest of the endocrine system is illustrated in Diagram 2. Emotional and psychological stress have their effect on the endocrine system via the hypothalamus.

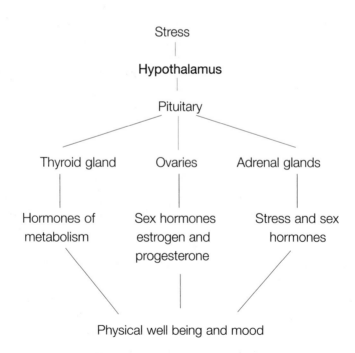

Diagram 2. The influence of stress on the endocrine system

24

The female menstrual cycle

Oestrogen and progesterone are the two hormones produced in the ovaries that control a woman's monthly cycle. Most women have heard of these, especially in connection with the contraceptive pill or with HRT. They do not work alone (nothing in nature is that simple!) but rather in harmony with two other hormones, follicle stimulating hormone (FSH) and luteinising hormone (LH). Just to add to the complex cycle there is also gonadotrophic hormone (GnRH) released by the hypothalamus to start the menstrual cycle off each month.

The cycle works on a cascade system from the hypothalamus to the ovaries via the pituitary, with one hormone stimulating the release of another, which in its turn suppresses the release of another. It goes something like this:

The hypothalamus releases GnRH

which stimulates the pituitary to release FSH and LH

which stimulates the ovaries to secrete progesterone and oestrogen

Diagram 3. Cascade effect of hormones during the menstrual cycle

Average monthly cycle

The average monthly cycle has hormones cascading over a 28-day cycle (remember that every women is different and not all follow the text book 28-day menstrual cycle).

Days 1 to between days 8 and 11 of the cycle (the follicular phase)

FSH causes an egg to develop in one of the ovaries and stimulates the ovaries to produce oestrogen to prepare for the release of an egg and to prepare the lining of the uterus (the endometrium) for receiving a fertilised egg. Oestrogen prepares a girl for puberty. Each girl is born with an estimated one million follicles (small egg sacs). Only around 400 reach full maturity. The rest degenerate at some point in their development with few follicles, if any, remaining at menopause.

Day 13

Oestrogen levels fall, sending a message to the pituitary to stop FSH production and increase LH production.

Day 14

Approximately 18 hours before ovulation occurs, LH levels soar stimulating the release of an egg into the fallopian tubes.

Days 15 to 25 (the luteal phase)

The corpus luteum (yellow body), formed from the follicle after the egg is released, secretes large quantities of progesterone to maintain the lining of the uterus ready for a pregnancy.

Day 26

When the egg is not fertilised, the corpus luteum degenerates which brings about a fall in both progesterone and oestrogen. The uterus lining breaks down.

Day 28

Menstruation starts

The next time you have a blood test, ask for a copy of the results and check your hormone levels against the reference ranges for different stages of the monthly cycle.

CHAPTER 4
YOUR HORMONES ONE BY ONE

For a woman to make informed choices about her health and medical treatments, she should have at least some idea of the workings of her own body and the possible impact of conventional medicine, particularly treatment for hormone problems. Most women have a fairly hazy knowledge about their reproductive hormones, namely oestrogen and progesterone, and their interaction with each other. I have therefore gone into some detail in this chapter about each of these hormones and included information about DHEA (dehydroepiandrosterone) because, as shown in diagram 4, so many other hormones can be made from DHEA.

Most people are surprised to discover that the 'female' hormones, oestrogen and progesterone, are not unique to women. Men produce these hormones too. For example, in the brain, testosterone is converted into oestrogen before it can be used to govern 'male' behaviour! Conversely, women produce small amounts of testosterone in the ovaries and adrenals which are converted into oestrogens. There are no uniquely male or female hormones, it is the concentration of the different hormones that governs whether we are male or female.

A simplified version of the manufacture of oestrogens, progesterone, testosterone and DHEA in the adrenal glands looks like this:

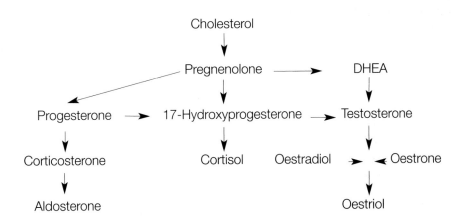

Diagram 4. Hormone production in the adrenal glands

Pregnenolone is the precursor to both progesterone and DHEA and the hormones corticosterone (important in the metabolism of glucose), aldosterone (needed for mineral metabolism) and cortisol (manufactured and released in response to stress), while oestrogens and testosterone can be made from both DHEA and progesterone.

What are oestrogen and progesterone?

Oestrogens and progesterone are steroid hormones and are part of a group of steroid hormones comprising cortisol, aldosterone, DHEA and testosterone. All the steroid hormones are manufactured from cholesterol – the fatty substance that has been much maligned in relation to cardiovascular disease, but without which your endocrine system would not function. The following is a profile of oestrogen, progesterone and DHEA, and how they work both individually and together as part of the endocrine system. I have also highlighted the differences between your own naturally produced hormones and those that are included in HRT (hormone replacement therapy).

More than one oestrogen

While people usually think of oestrogen as one hormone, there are in fact three main types of oestrogen, oestrone (E1), oestradiol (E2) and oestriol (E3), with at least another two dozen different kinds.

Oestrogens have more than three hundred functions in the body. For example, in the brain oestrogens are requred for verbal learning and to enhance the capacity to learn new ideas, to reduce cholesterol levels in the blood, to ensure adequate calcium in the bones, and to increase the production of collagen and elastin (both required for keeping the skin hydrated and elastic.)[16] Oestrogen is also involved in immune function where too high levels have been linked with auto-immune diseases such as endometriosis, Hashimoto's thyroiditis, systemic lupus erythermatosus, Sjogren's disease, Grave's disease, and rheumatoid arthritis.[17]

Oestradiol is the most powerful and the most dominant form of oestrogen in a non-pregnant woman. Produced mainly in the ovaries, oestradiol is converted in the liver and small intestine to oestrone and then into oestriol. When a woman is not pregnant, oestriol is produced in small quantities with oestradiol predominating. During pregnancy, oestriol levels rise and it becomes the predominant form of oestrogen, along with soaring levels of progesterone.[18]

Oestrone and breast cancer

Oestrone is thought to be more carcinogenic than oestradiol or oestriol, and is the form of oestrogen most responsible for breast cancer. The most commonly prescribed oral HRT contains oestrone or oestradiol, or a combination of the two hormones. However, as oestradiol is converted to oestrone in the liver and intestines, this means that most orally administered HRT is, in effect, oestrone.[19]

The importance of B vitamins, fibre and gut flora

Oestriol is a benign form of oestrogen and is also the form in which the body is able to successfully excrete oestrogens once they have done their job. The liver is dependent on a plentiful supply of B vitamins, including choline and inositol, to carry out the conversion of oestradiol and oestrone to oestriol ready for excretion. If there are insufficient B vitamins in the diet, oestradiol/oestrone levels can remain too high, leading to changes in breast tissue, the occurrence of breast cancer and endometriosis.[20]

In the intestines, oestriol is bound to fibre and excreted via the colon – providing there is enough fibre available. A diet low in fibre and high in fat (particularly processed and animal fats), changes the ability of the gut flora (beneficial intestinal bacteria) to break down oestrogens effectively.

When normal gut flora are disrupted, instead of oestrogens being properly eliminated, they can be reactivated as oestrone and reabsorbed into the bloodstream. This leads to an overall rise in levels of oestrone in relation to oestradiol and oestriol. To a lesser extent this will cause period problems and PMS, fibroids and cysts, and at the other extreme it can lead to breast cancer.

It's therefore easy to see how fibre, B vitamins, the right kinds of fats and the presence of balanced intestinal (gut) flora are all vital components in balancing hormones naturally. In part two of this book you will find out how to balance your diet in favour of fibre, B vitamins and gut flora.

Oestriol prevents and protects against breast cancer

Oestradiol and oestrone are used in conventional HRT preparations, despite the fact that they are known to cause breast cancer. Yet research shows that the benign form of oestrogen, oestriol, not only protects against breast cancer, it has even been shown to reverse the disease!

Much of the research into the beneficial effects of oestriol has been carried out by Dr. H. M. Lemon and associates at the University of Nebraska.[21, 22] Dr. Lemon found that women with breast cancer have low levels of oestriol relative to the other forms of oestrogen when compared with women who did not have breast cancer. He showed that oestriol therapy can in fact inhibit breast cancer. Even postmenopausal women whose breast cancer had metastised (spread), experienced a remission or arrest of metastatic lesions with oestriol therapy.

In "*Estrogen Replacement Therapy. Excerpted from Preventing and Reversing Osteoporosis*", Alan R. Gaby, M.D. points out that conventional oestrogen therapy can cause a potentially precancerous proliferation of the uterine lining, known as endometrial hyperplasia. By contrast most investigators have found that oestriol does not cause endometrial proliferation.[23]

Oestriol available on prescription

Although oestrogen production in the ovaries decreases with the menopause, it continues to be produced in the adrenals from progesterone or from androgens (male hormones), particularly from DHEA (see diagram 4). However, for women with a proven medical need for oestrogen, natural oestriol is available on prescription and it is certainly worth talking to your doctor about this alternative. According to Alan Gaby, M.D., a dose of 2 to 4 mg of oestriol is considered equivalent to, and as effective as, 0.6 to 1.25 mg of conjugated oestrogens or oestrone.

But why not increase oestrogen levels naturally? Yes, it can be done!

Vitamin E

Vitamin E is a powerful anti-oxidant that protects fats in the diet and in the cells and helps protect against cancer. But it seems that it isn't just its antioxidant activity that makes vitamin E so useful in hormone treatments. It has also been shown to increase oestriol levels in the blood. Women with fibrocystic breast disease (fibrocystic breast disease is believed to increase a woman's risk of breast cancer) who took 600 i.u.s per day of vitamin E were found to have an 18% increase in the ratio of oestriol to oestradiol. If vitamin E increases oestriol levels, it shows that there is more to vitamin E's anti-cancer properties than just being an antioxidant.[24,25]

Boron

Boron, a mineral found to be essential for strong bones and the prevention of osteoporosis, has its effect on bones through its ability to naturally raise oestrogen levels in the blood, particularly a form of oestradiol. However, it also increases levels of oestriol in the blood. Taking around 1 - 3 mg of boron per day is sufficient and all good multi vitamin and mineral supplements should contain boron, especially if they are aimed at women.[26]

Phytoestrogens

Phytoestrogens, the weak hormones found in all foods of plant origin, but particularly high in linseeds, seaweed, and fermented soya products, block the effect of environmental oestrogens and help naturally balance a woman's own hormone production (see chapter two).

Progesterone

Progesterone is produced in the ovaries and is the hormone most dominant during the second half of the menstrual cycle. Its functions are to make changes to the endometrial lining (the lining of the uterus) in preparation for receiving a fertilised egg and, in effect, to act as a counter balance to oestrogen. Levels of progesterone increase dramatically during pregnancy when it is produced by the placenta to maintain a healthy pregnancy.

As oestrogen levels in the ovaries decline during the menopause, the production of progesterone from mature eggs also declines and eventually stops altogether. However, like oestrogens, progesterone will continue to be produced from cholesterol, via pregnenolone, in the adrenals after menopause. Diagram 4 shows how progesterone can be used in the adrenal cortex to manufactre DHEA, testosterone and oestrogens, as well as corticosterone, aldosterone and cortisol.

Stress reduces progesterone levels

Because of the interlinking of the steroid hormones, including the stress hormone, cortisol, stress can have a big impact on the amount of progesterone available in the body. Not only does stress cause a rise in cortisol levels which block progesterone receptor sites in cells, but cortisol can also compete with progesterone for production from pregnenolone. Women displaying symptoms of hormone distress are usually suffering from a number of different forms of stress, including emotional, physical, environmental and nutritional. All this stress can add up to a reduction in progesterone levels, and a subsequent rise in oestrogen levels, leading to oestrogen dominance.

Oestrogen or progesterone deficient?

Many symptoms normally treated medically as an oestrogen deficiency may in fact be due to an overall imbalance in oestrogen/progesterone, with oestrogen in dominance. If symptoms diminish using natural progesterone, this indicates that lack of progesterone rather oestrogen deficiency may be the cause of the symptoms.

In menstruating women symptoms of hormonal distress include :

- Anovulatory menstrual cycles, i.e. no ovulation, making it more difficult to conceive
- Premenstrual syndrome
- Weight gain
- Menstrual cycle irregularity
- Infertility
- Endometriosis
- Fibroids
- Fibrocystic breast disease
- Uterine and breast cancer
- Abnormal thyroid function

During the years leading up to the menopause, as progesterone levels start to naturally decline, women suffer from a wide range of symptoms that are usually all lumped under the heading "menopause". They include :

- Hot flushes
- Insomnia
- Night sweats
- Weight gain
- Loss of libido
- Water retention (bloating)
- Vaginal itching, soreness and drying leading to pain during intercourse
- Mood swings, irritability , depression, anxiety and panic attacks
- Osteoporosis

A more complete list of symptoms can be found in Chapters 6 and 7.

Is the answer to take progesterone?

The question of hormone replacement therapy (HRT) is discussed more fully in chapter 7. However, before you start supplementing your own hormones with any form of hormone replacement, please read the rest of this section.

Progesterone v. progestogens

It is important to understand the difference between progesterone naturally produced by the body and the synthetic progestogen (progestin in the U.S.) used in hormone medication. Progestogen, for example medroxyprogesterone acetate found in Provera, is a molecularly modified version of progesterone and is not identical to anything found in nature.

Progestogens occupy the receptor sites normally occupied by the body's own progesterone, blocking progesterone from carrying out its normal functions.

For example, progesterone reverses the cancer-causing effects of oestrogen. It does this by slowing breast cell proliferation through its action on the p53 gene, the gene associated with DNA damage and cancer. Progestogen cannot do this and gets in the way of progesterone's natural protective activity.[27]

While progesterone is needed for a viable and healthy pregnancy, progestogen can cause birth defects and should not be used during pregnancy.

Progestogen is used in hormone preparations such as the Pill and HRT to counter the effects of oestrogen, but does not show up in blood or saliva tests. This is because it is not raising levels of progesterone in the body.

Documented side effects from taking progestogens include:

• Depression, nausea, insomnia or sleepiness
• Skin sensitivity such as itching and skin rashes
• Acne, alopecia (hair loss) and hirsuitism (male pattern hair growth)
• Cervical erosions and changes in cervical secretions
• Severe allergic reactions
• Thrombophlebitis and pulmonary embolism
• Fluid retention (oedema) and weight changes
• Loss of sex drive
• Rise in temperature
• Ovarian cysts
• Break-through bleeding and spotting
• Menstrual irregularity
• Epilepsy, migraine, asthma
• Cardiac or renal dysfunction
• Increased risk of birth defects (should not be used during pregnancy)
• Reduced milk production
• Bloating, abdominal cramps, anxiety and irritability[28]
• Breast tenderness, increased risk of breast cancer
• Reduced HDL (the good cholesterol)
• Increased risk of thrombembolism (blood clots)
• Changes in glucose and insulin levels
• Higher than normal levels of calcium in the blood
• Liver cancer, jaundice[29]
• Increased risk for coronary heart disease, invasive breast cancer, stroke, pulmonary embolism, endometrial cancer, colorectal cancer, hip fracture[30]

Natural progesterone

Natural progesterone, more accurately called 'botanical or nature identical', is manufactured in a laboratory from either wild yam or soya. Public awareness of natural progesterone and the dangers of progestogens is due to Dr. John Lee, an American M.D., who has been using natural progesterone for many years in his practice in America, with good results. Dr. Lee has used natural progesterone to treat all kinds of hormone-related health problems caused by too high levels of oestrogen (oestrogen dominance), including osteoporosis. He has numerous anecdotal patient case studies showing a reversal of osteoporosis using a combination of natural progesterone, exercise, a good diet and natural food supplements (see chapter 8).

In his Medical Letter, "*Study shows breast cancer risk for women using HRT*" dated February 2000, Dr. Lee even goes as far as to state, "*Prescribing a progestin to a menopausal woman should be considered medical malpractice!*"

In her book, "*Natural alternatives to HRT*", Marilyn Glenville comes down heavily against the use of progesterone, natural or otherwise. Her argument says that natural progesterone is not natural at all but synthesised in a laboratory, usually from soya. Women naturally stop producing progesterone once they reach menopause so there should be no need to supplement this hormone.[31]

In an ideal world where women are not stressed and are eating a perfectly balanced diet high in mineral-rich plant material, where there is no pollution and no synthetic hormones leading to oestrogen dominance, there would be no need to supplement with natural progesterone. Unfortunately we live in a world where oestrogen dominance is a fact of life in both our external and internal environments. Women are stressed and trying to do too much, they do not eat a well balanced diet and they are taking hormones both as medication and in food. All this leads to a decline in progesterone levels in women any time after their mid-thirties that continues through menopause.

As hormone dependent cancers are usually due to oestrogen dominance, and therefore progesterone deficiency, breast cancer is often diagnosed in women in their late forties and early fifties, following ten years or so of progesterone deficiency. Supplementing with natural progesterone can help prevent the development of cancer, as well as reducing the symptoms of both PMS and menopause.[32]

How 'natural' is natural progesterone?

On the question of whether natural progesterone is natural or not, Dr. Lee states that natural progesterone, while synthesised in a laboratory, has the identical molecular configuration of the progesterone made in the body. It is *"nature identical"* to your own progesterone. Conversely, progestogens are made from the same plant source as nature identical progesterone, but the molecular structure is changed so that it is unlike anything found in nature.[33]

Cream or pills?

Natural progesterone comes in two forms: a transdermal cream (rubbed into the skin) and micronised oral progesterone (taken as a pill). Oral progesterone is more commonly prescribed by doctors in Europe than progesterone cream, although Dr. Lee recommends progesterone cream rather than oral progesterone because oral progesterone has to go via the liver where between 80% and 90% is broken down and lost. Because of this loss, at least 200 to 400 mg daily is needed to achieve a physiologic dose of 15 - 24 mg (a normally menstruating woman produces between 20 and 30 mg per day during the second {luteal} phase of her cycle). Such high doses create undesirable metabolites or biochemical by-products that can unnecessarily overload the liver, the body's main organ for detoxification.

Measuring progesterone levels

Levels of hormones in the blood can be measured with a blood or saliva test, but these can give different results. According to Dr. Lee, blood tests for progesterone measure the plasma concentration of progesterone (plasma is the clear liquid part of the blood after all the red and white blood cells have been removed) and only pick up 2% to 5% of "free" or bioavailable progesterone. The remaining progesterone is on its way back to the liver for excretion in the bile and is not destined for use by the body. On the other hand, progesterone transported in red blood cells is available for use in all the target tissues and in saliva.[34]

Saliva testing has been found to be a much more accurate test for bioavailable levels of progesterone in the blood following application of progesterone cream. Dr. Lee states that the timing between applying the cream and doing the saliva test is crucial because there is a peak of progesterone concentration in the blood two or three hours after application of the cream, after which it is metabolised and excreted by the liver. The time it takes to be metabolised and excreted depends on the health of a woman's liver. If the cream is being applied twice a day, then saliva collection should be about 10 hours after application. However, if it is being applied just once a day, then saliva collection should be 24 hours after the previous application.[35]

Can you have too much of a good thing?

Women who are using natural progesterone cream, thinking it is the panacea for all their hormone-related problems, should make sure not to exceed the directions for use, especially if they are tempted to think that more is better. With saliva testing, there is evidence that women using oral progesterone and 10% strength progesterone cream (both available on prescription only) can develop a progesterone excess as it builds up in the fat layer under the skin. Symptoms of excess progesterone can start with lethargy and depression and then go on to mimic the very symptoms progesterone therapy was trying to correct in the first place.[36]

Apparently this problem does not occur in women using over the counter 3% progesterone cream, providing they use it at the recommended dose of 1/8 to 1/4 of a teaspoon once or twice a day, depending on severity of symptoms. A 1/4 teaspoon supplies approximately 20 mg of progesterone. Menstruating women should use it between days 12 and 26 of their cycle. Menopausal women should use it for three weeks on, one week off. It is applied to soft tissue areas of the body where blood vessels are close to the skin, such as inner arms and thighs, breasts and abdominal area. As only about 60% of anything applied to the skin is absorbed, these recommended doses should avoid a build up of progesterone in the body.

Where to obtain natural progesterone cream

Natural progesterone is available on prescription in Europe and the UK as oral progesterone, or as a gel or cream.

In the U.S. natural progesterone cream is freely available over the counter in pharmacies and health food stores and via the internet.

Improving nutrition first

All hormones, natural or otherwise, should be used with caution to avoid upsetting the body's own balance. Often optimum nutrition and nutritional supplements can achieve hormone balance without resorting to hormone preparations. However, in certain health problems such as osteoporosis, endometriosis, infertility, fast growing fibroids and hormone-related cancers, natural progesterone can be an important part of a natural approach to healing. Natural progesterone can also help ease the transition through menopause by reducing symptoms and helping maintain a feeling of equilibrium (see chapter 8).

DHEA

DHEA (dehydroepiandrosterone) is an androgen (male hormone) manufactured from cholesterol in the adrenals. As well as being closely involved in controlling glucose levels and in stimulating immune function, DHEA is also converted to oestrogens and testosterone. Its function is similar to that of pregnenolone and has been called the 'mother of all hormones'.

DHEA levels reach their peak between the ages of 20 and 30, and then decrease dramatically over the next five to six decades, losing around 10% of their value per decade. As well as naturally decreasing with age, DHEA levels are lowered by high insulin levels where its role in lowering insulin causes it to be diverted from its other functions. DHEA is also decreased as a result of extreme stress as cortisol production competes with the production of DHEA.

Fountain of youth?

In postmenopausal women much of the continuing oestrogen production in the adrenals may come from DHEA. Because of this it has been touted as a fountain of youth and in America supplements of DHEA are freely available over the counter. In Europe, DHEA is only available on prescription. Jeffrey S. Bland, PhD, nutritional biochemist and pioneer in the field of functional medicine, advises caution when using DHEA therapeutically. While in premenopausal women DHEA can inhibit cancerous tumours, the opposite is true in postmenopausal women where DHEA can stimulate the growth of breast cancer cells.[36]

Maintaining DHEA naturally

DHEA is available on prescription where levels have fallen very low and are leading to extreme fatigue and adrenal exhaustion. However, you can encourage the adrenals to continue producing sufficient DHEA by avoiding foods that cause the stimulation of insulin secretion, particularly sugar, caffeine, cocoa and chocolate, alcohol and highly salted foods.

In addition, a healthy diet high in B vitamins, zinc, calcium and magnesium, vitamin C and omega-3 fatty acids, combined with supplements to provide extra nutrients during times of stress, will also help your adrenals to function normally.

Ginseng and liquorice are both remedies for encouraging the natural production of DHEA and are available in teas and in supplements.

CHAPTER 5
THE MENSTRUATING YEARS

Premenstrual syndrome

During the menstruating years, the most common problem that affects women is PMS (premenstrual syndrome) – formerly called PMT or premenstrual tension. The name 'premenstrual syndrome' acknowledges the wide ranging number of symptoms that can occur with this condition. The symptoms can vary widely in severity and duration from one woman to the next, and from one month to the next.

The majority of women who consult me, whether for PMS specifically or for other health problems, suffer from some degree of PMS. Those who don't mention it as a problem have just assumed that it is normal to feel lousy, irritable, have pain and be miserable around period time. PMS is such a common phenomenon for so many women (usually affecting those close to them as well), that it may come as a surprise to learn that while it has become normal, it is not natural. You do not have to suffer with it!

What is premenstrual syndrome?

A syndrome is a collection of symptoms and in the case of PMS can range through the physical, psychological and emotional, often including them all. If you experience any of the following between one and fourteen days before two out of three periods, you are likely to be suffering from PMS:

Physical symptoms

Water retention; breast tenderness and swelling; weight gain; abdominal cramps and bloating; migraines/headaches; acne; backache; excessive thirst; insomnia; food cravings (especially sweet foods); lack of co-ordination; fatigue; lack of energy; lack of concentration; forgetfulness; dizziness; susceptibility to infection.

Emotional symptoms

Depression; confusion; mood swings; irritability; tension and anxiety; panic attacks; aggressive behaviour; tearfulness; suicidal thoughts (seek help immediately if you have these).

Trudy's story

Trudy consulted me with severe PMS which started a week before her period was due. Symptoms included bloating, fatigue, irritability, depression, breast tenderness, headaches and mood swings so bad that her family ran for cover. Other symptoms included acne, cravings for sweet things, heavy periods, splitting nails, eczema, irritable bowel syndrome and abdominal cramping. Her blood tests were perfectly normal for hormonal balance. Treatment using the Pill had been unsuccessful in her case, causing high blood pressure and weight gain.

From the questionnaire that I had asked Trudy to fill in and from our consultation, I identified the following probable causes of her symptoms:

- A leaky gut (when the intestinal membrane becomes over permeable)
- Low stomach acid
- Poor elimination due to lack of fibre, exercise and water
- Blood sugar fluctuations with hypoglycaemia (low blood sugar)
- Food intolerances
- Nutritional deficiencies right across the board, including B vitamins, zinc, calcium, magnesium and selenium

I decided to concentrate on improving her digestion, absorption and elimination, cutting out nutritional stressors such as caffeine, sugar and alcohol, and avoiding dairy produce. I gave her quite a lengthy list of supplements to take initially, which caused some consternation among family and friends.

A delighted Trudy lost 3 kg (half a stone) within two months and her periods were very much lighter with less PMS. Stopping some of the supplements too soon caused her symptoms to reappear very quickly. Returning to the full programme for a further three months brought about improvement in her skin, a complete clearing up of the eczema and lighter, more regular periods. Trudy discovered the joy of having a normal period each month with no PMS and only a slight feeling of fatigue on the first day. Nothing else.

Trudy still takes a maintenance supplement programme and is now able to self indulge on occasions without her health suffering as a result.

What causes PMS ?

Premenstrual syndrome implies a certain degree of hormone distress or imbalance, although an imbalance is rarely picked up on a blood test. Because the endocrine system is so interlinked, an imbalance in one area can throw the rest out of kilter (see chapter 3).

Lowered progesterone levels

The most common cause of PMS is a too high ratio of oestrogen to progesterone. According to Kate Neil and Patrick Holford in their book, "*Balancing Hormones Naturally*", 75% of all PMS sufferers fall into this category. Environmentally, women's hormones are being disrupted by xenoestrogens found in petrochemical derivatives used as herbicides and pesticides, in food packaging and as industrial fallout, hormone medication and in the water supply. This is contributing to raised oestrogen and lowered progesterone levels. Only a small minority have higher levels of progesterone to oestrogen.

Stress

Hormone disharmony is being caused by the stress of women trying to do too much, getting insufficient rest, relaxation, sleep and time for self. Women are also spending too much time sitting at a desk, inside in artificial lighting and often breathing recycled air. They are not getting enough exercise or exposure to fresh air and sunshine. Too much stress leads to high levels of cortisol which depress progesterone levels

Blood sugar control

The level of stimulants consumed by most women causes disglycaemia (erratic fluctuations in blood sugar control) leading to alternating bouts of hyperglycaemia and hypoglycaemia (high and low blood sugar). The symptoms of low blood sugar very closely resemble the symptoms of PMS. The stimulants that cause disglycaemia include caffeine, sugar and sugary foods, chocolate, alcohol, salty foods and snacks, and nicotine (see chapter 11).

The trouble with stimulants is that periods of hypoglycaemia cause cravings for yet more stimulants, sometimes so severe that women feel irritable, depressed, aggressive and incapable of functioning properly until the craving has been satisfied. Cutting the cycle of highs and lows in energy levels and cravings is the only way to achieve more energy, less fatigue and a balance in hormone function.

Chromium, manganese, zinc and vitamins B6 and B3 are required for insulin production and blood sugar control. They are heavily depleted in foods that have been refined as all the vitamins and minerals are found in the germ of seeds and grains and just under the skin in vegetables, i.e. potatoes. Women who are consuming a diet high in processed foods and stimulants can soon become deficient in nutrients needed for stable blood sugar. In sensitive women, a continued over-stimulation of insulin production may eventually lead to diabetes.

Nutritional deficiencies

Women are eating more processed foods and suffering from nutritional deficiencies as a result. The lack of fibre, the wrong kind of fats, lack of B vitamins, zinc and essential fatty acids, combined with too many stimulants, are causing too much circulating oestrogen and a lack of progesterone.

Vitamin B6 and the B vitamins

Several studies have looked at the effects of vitamin B6 on premenstrual syndrome symptoms. Researchers in Oxford showed that 50 mg of vitamin B6 per day had a significant beneficial effect on emotional symptoms such as depression, irritability and tiredness.[38] Vitamin B6 is necessary for the production of serotonin and dopamine, and a deficiency may lead to or aggravate the effects of PMS through effects on these neurotransmitters.

As well as being important for converting oestrogens in the liver for excretion, B vitamins also affect brain chemistry, energy production and blood sugar control where they are needed for insulin production. A lack of B vitamins leads to low energy, irritability, mood swings and depression.

Magnesium

Red blood cell concentrations of magnesium are low in women with PMS, the most common symptom of magnesium deficiency being period pain and cramping. However, magnesium is required in the production of energy so a lack of it will lead to low energy levels. Taking vitamin B6 with magnesium raises magnesium levels in red blood cells. The calcium to magnesium ratio also seems to be affected by hormonal fluctuations, which may affect neurotransmitter levels and lead to premenstrual symptoms.[39,40] I have found magnesium supplementation in the form of magnesium citrate very effective at relieving some of the symptoms of PMS.

42

Calcium

Calcium works with magnesium and is important in nerve transmission. Sufficient calcium leads to a feeling of calm. A 1998 study showed that during the luteal (second half) phase of the menstrual cycle, women who took calcium experienced significantly fewer symptoms than those who did not. Mood swings and depression were reduced by 45 per cent (compared to 28 per cent in the placebo group), while generalized aches and pains, back pains and cramping reduced by 54 per cent in three months.[41]

Vitamin E

Vitamin E reduces breast tenderness and other symptoms of PMS by raising levels of oestriol, the benign form of oestrogen that has been shown to protect against breast cancer. Reducing caffeine and alcohol consumption also helps relieve breast tenderness. Refined foods and oils have lost all their vitamin E. Best sources are whole grains, seeds and nuts.[42]

Zinc

Zinc is an important component of hormone production. Zinc and copper are balanced in the body with a deficiency of zinc leading to an excess of copper. Zinc deficiency leads to a lack of progesterone in the second half of the menstrual cycle. The Pill also causes zinc deficiency and an excess of copper. Women who suffer from PMS are invariably zinc deficient.[43] The highest food source of zinc are fresh oysters, which is why they have a reputation for being an aphrodisiac. Zinc's influence on hormones means that it indirectly influences libido. Zinc is better absorbed from meat and fish, but nuts, eggs and pulses (dried beans, peas and lentils) are also a good source of zinc.

Essential fatty acids

Essential fatty acids are the kind of fats that the body needs to produce and transport hormones in the blood. They are found in all whole, unprocessed foods, particularly in seeds, oily fish and cold pressed oils. Processed fats found in all bakery products contain a high level of trans fatty acids which interfere with the conversion and absorption of essential fatty acids in the body.

Alcohol also blocks essential fatty acid utilisation and many women experience relief from PMS symptoms when they switch to cold pressed oils, eat seeds and stop drinking alcohol. Taking a supplement of essential fatty acids from evening primrose oil, borage oil, blackcurrant oil and linseed oil can very quickly help to relieve PMS, the pain of breast tenderness and abdominal cramping.[44]

Losing touch with the inner woman

I believe a lot of women have lost touch with themselves as part of the cycle of nature and with both their physical and emotional needs. In an effort to get on in a man's world, women have become separated from their innate wisdom and are forgetting to look after themselves through their diet, rest, exercise, sleep and spiritual nourishment. Doing too much leads to feeling overwhelmed and unable to cope – classic signs of stress. I see enough stressed and burnt out men to know that it's not a bed of roses for the average man trying to survive in a modern working environment, but how often have you heard a man being asked how he manages to combine work and family life?

Countless polls reported in the media show that, no matter how much more modern men are doing (or think they do) in the home, it is still women who take on the major burden of running the home and taking care of the kids, as well as working full time. If you add the impact of environmental pollution onto a pressurised lifestyle, then it's hardly surprising so many women wonder if it is worth being female at all !

Ask for help

Single parents experience even higher levels of stress and stress-related hormone disruption. For them the pressure is extreme because there is no one with whom they can share the burden. In that case excellent nutrition and supplements can help women deal with the extra stress of managing alone. And if help is available, don't be afraid to ask. Traditionally women formed their own support groups helping each other out when times got tough. Now, with so many women working outside the home according to male working practices, this support has become fragmented and women can feel isolated. Whatever your stage in life, but particularly if you are struggling with ill health, a young family and a full time job, establishing female support can be really helpful in reducing stress levels.

The Pill as treatment for hormone imbalance

Whatever the underlying causes, hormones in the form of the Pill are routinely prescribed to treat PMS, especially where there is pain and/or heavy bleeding. Taking the Pill can provide a huge relief for some women and many find their symptoms do get better. Unfortunately, the treatment deals with the symptoms but does not get to the root cause of the problem, so that when the prescribed hormones are discontinued for any reason, the problems return – often more severely.

In addition, synthetic hormones compete for receptor sites normally available to home produced hormones and they overload the body with standard measurements of molecularly modified hormones that may be more than the body can deal with fast enough.

Many of the women who come to see me do so because they have not had any success with the Pill or they are afraid of the increased risk of cancer due to taking hormones. Women report side effects from the Pill that include headaches, weight gain, mood swings, depression, insomnia, breast lumps and break-through bleeding (see Irene's story in the Introduction). Those who do feel better with the Pill understandably do not want to give up their hormone treatment. They are afraid of returning to the state of hormonal health that existed before they started the treatment.

Long term side effects of using the Pill

Taking oestrogen causes cancer. The Pill contains a mixture of oestrogen and progestogens, both of which are now known to cause cancer. There have been many studies over the years highlighting the link between taking hormones and increased rates of hormone-related cancers, i.e. breast, uterine, endometrial, cervical and ovarian cancer. As long ago as 1986, Dr. Ellen Grant, an enthusiastic advocate of the Pill in the 1960s, was warning of the dangers in taking the Pill in her book, "*The Bitter Pill*". She says, "*It is impossible to estimate the real cost of treating or alleviating the illness, social tragedies and handicaps that have been caused by the Pill. No British government would now hand out free cigarettes, and yet the Pill causes as much illness as smoking.*" [45]

Increased rates of cancer

A number of women have asked me if the danger of cancer only applies to the older generation of higher dose Pill. Research shows that the modern lower dose Pill is just as harmful. A study presented to the third European Breast Cancer conference in Barcelona in March 2002, with research carried out by Dr. Merethe Kumle and her team from the Institute of Community Medicine in Tromso, Norway, reported an increased risk of 26% for breast cancer in women who had used the Pill at any time in their lives. Women who had used the Pill over longer periods of time increased their risk of breast cancer by 58% compared with those who had never used it, with the highest increased risk (144%) among women aged over 45 who were still using the Pill. The study used data collected from 103,027 Norwegian and Swedish women who were questioned about their lifestyle, health and use of the Pill in 1991/1992.

Most of the women who had taken the Pill had used the more modern brands that are currently prescribed by doctors. Dr. Kumle states in her report to the Barcelona conference, *"It is clear that oral contraceptives increase a woman's risk of developing breast cancer, particularly when they are used in the later period of reproductive life."*[46]

Alternatives to the Pill

Optimum nutrition offers a very effective alternative to the Pill for the treatment of PMS and problems with periods, such as period irregularity or infrequency, heavy bleeding and/or pain. Numbers of women call me just two to three weeks after starting their nutrition programme to say that their next period has arrived with either vastly reduced symptoms, or no symptoms at all. The effect can be that quick. Sometimes I recommend using herbs as well as vitamins, minerals, essential fatty acids and change of diet. All of this is discussed in chapter 15.

Reversing hormone imbalance

Reversing hormonal imbalance involves all of the following:

- Rebalance the diet with healthy, natural foods high in fibre, with complex carbohydrates, good quality protein, and a predominance of fruit and vegetables for their high phytohormone content (chapter 11)

- Correct poor blood sugar control (chapter 13)

- Improve digestion, absorption and elimination (chapter 14)

- Treat candidiasis if it is a contributing factor (chapter 6)

- Check for the existence of food allergies (chapter 7)

- Check for low thyroid function (chapter 8)

- Make up the shortfall in nutritional deficiencies (chapter 15)

- Use herbal and plant-based remedies where appropriate (chapter 15)

- Avoid environmental oestrogens and hormone medication where at all possible (chapter 2)

- Make time for yourself to rest, relax and take some exercise and fresh air. When the sun shines, get outside and enjoy it. So many people miss daily fresh air and sun because they work through their lunchtimes. It is important to take a break in the middle of the day and go outside and walk. Breaking up the day means you will feel less tired and stale in the afternoon. A change of scenery is also a very good way of de-stressing if you have had a pressurised morning.

• Remember to breathe! Next time you are rushing around, feeling tense, getting into an argument with your partner, colleague or boss, check your breathing. Most people hold their breath or breathe very shallowly when they are under stress. Try stopping whatever you are doing and take a deep breath that really fills the lungs. When you inflate your lungs properly, your diaphragm and abdominal area will go out. Hold this breath for the count of three and then let it out slowly. Repeat the process three times. If you feel a bit dizzy, it's because you have just given your brain a dose of oxygen after it has been deprived for some time. Check in at regular intervals during the day and notice what your breath is doing.

• Ask for help and support and don't expect to be Superwoman!

Whether you are suffering from PMS or fibroids, endometriosis or breast cancer, making nutritional and lifestyle changes will help your hormones find their own balance and give your body a chance to heal itself.

CHAPTER 6
THE CANDIDA CONNECTION

Candidiasis syndrome

Candidiasis, often simply referred to as 'candida', is the name given to a syndrome that describes a wide range of symptoms associated with systemic fungal or yeast infection, which can have a profound effect on all systems of the body, affecting both physical and mental health.

What is candida?

We all have living within our colons 1.5 - 2 kg of bacteria (our gut flora), yeasts and other micro-organisms. Some of these bacteria, the bifidus bacteria, are beneficial and carry out some very useful biochemical reactions, including the production of antibiotics and some vitamins, and processing hormones ready for excretion. Other inhabitants of our intestines, the pathogenic bacteria and yeasts, are not useful at all and can be positively harmful. This is not something to be concerned about under normal circumstances provided the balance is tipped in favour of the beneficial kind.

Of the yeasts, candida albicans (one of a family of candida yeasts) is the one most commonly involved in fungal and yeast infections. When the good bacteria become suppressed, the yeasts have a chance to proliferate and get out of control, causing many of the health problems associated with candidiasis. Factors known to favour candida because they either suppress good bacteria or the immune system, or they 'feed' the yeast are :

- Antibiotics
- Steroid medication
- Hormone medication (Pill or HRT)
- Hormonal changes e.g. puberty, sexual maturity, pregnancy, sterilisation, menopause
- Amalgam fillings (silver fillings contain mercury)
- Chemical poisoning in the home or office
- Stress, including noise pollution
- Immunisation (vaccinations) including infant immunisation (some vaccines contain a mercury derivative as a preservative)
- High sugar and alcohol consumption

Digestive problems

If the overgrowth of candida remains in the digestive tract the main problems will be digestive disruption, including abdominal bloating, pain, constipation and/or diarrhoea, indigestion, flatulence, belching and anal itching. If it moves further up the digestive tract sufferers experience fungal infections in the mouth (oral thrush) or constant sore throats and infections that may lead to more serious chest infections. Patients suffering with digestive problems that have no obvious cause are often told they have IBS (irritable bowel syndrome).

Changing identity from yeast to fungus

If the diet is deficient in biotin, one of the B vitamins, then the yeast can change into its mycelial or fungal form with the ability to put down hyphae (little root like projections) through the intestinal membrane, much like mould penetrating a piece of stale bread, and move into the blood. Once in the bloodstream, the fungus can travel around the body affecting any susceptible area (joints, muscles, organs, soft tissue and even the brain where it influences mood and mental well being).[47]

Poor digestion

With candida in the digestive tract, digestion of food is usually compromised. Insufficient stomach acid is produced to break down protein into its smallest components, and digestive enzymes secreted from the pancreas and gall bladder are unable to completely break down carbohydrates and fats. This means that incompletely digested food particles are reaching the intestines for absorption. The lining of the intestinal tract is designed to allow digested food particles such as amino acids, simple carbohydrates and lipid molecules through into the bloodstream for distribution around the body.

Leaky gut and allergies

As candida penetrates the intestinal membrane, it has the effect of making the intestinal membrane too 'holey', a bit like a colander instead of a sieve. This has graphically been termed 'leaky gut'. The improperly digested food particles are able to pass through these extra large holes into the bloodstream, where they are treated as alien substances by the immune system. This in turn leads to allergies and sensitivities, not just to many different foods, but also to outside agents such as pollen, house dust mite, animals, chemicals, petrol fumes, perfumes, cigarette smoke, etc.[48,49]

As the ability to digest and break down food for absorption is affected by the presence of candida, sufferers may find themselves becoming increasingly sensitive to a wide range of perfectly normal healthy foods. A vicious cycle sets in based on food intolerance, leaky gut, candidiasis and hormone disruption. Breaking the cycle is the only route back to hormone harmony. In chapter 7 you will find allergies and food intolerance explained in more detail, including instructions on how to carry out a simple and effective allergy test yourself at home.

Affinity with hormones

Candida has an affinity with hormones and is attracted to the endocrine system where it can cause most disruption. According to Dr. Christine Tomlinson (an ex-sufferer of candidiasis) of the U.K. National Candida Society[50], candida binds to circulating hormones, changing their shape so they are unable to attach to the receptor sites on the target cells. This effectively inactivates the hormone, stopping it from doing its job.

Women have a cyclical hormone pattern resulting in highs and lows of oestrogen and progesterone through the month, which is very appealing to candida. This is why there are more female sufferers than male, although men certainly do get it and over the years I have treated many men with candida infestation.

Symptoms most commonly associated with candida are thrush (vaginal and oral yeast infection), cystitis and fungal infections of the nails or skin (such as athlete's foot), digestive problems, PMS and menstrual irregularities. But as candida can also disrupt adrenal and thyroid function, symptoms can be many and varied and include joint pains, allergies, asthma, hayfever, muscle fatigue, chronic fatigue, exhaustion, blood sugar fluctuations and low thyroid function (often characterised by feeling cold).

Endocrine breakdown (APICH)

I have treated a number of both men and women suffering from the affects of complete endocrine disruption caused by candida. Blood tests show all hormone levels to be below normal ranges, and those people feel just terrible, suffering from extreme fatigue and exhaustion, muscle and joint pain, depression and lethargy. Women in particular suffer from PMS, menopausal symptoms, and often cysts and fibroids. Rather than feeling well within a matter of weeks, sufferers usually take several months and up to a year on an anti-candida nutrition programme before they start to recover. However, they do recover and go on to feel energetic and well.

This extreme reaction to candida has been identified by Endocrinologist Phyllis Saifer, M.D as APICH syndrome (autoimmune polyendocripopathy immune-dysregulation candidosis hypersensitivity syndrome).[51] This means that through the interaction between the endocrine and immune systems, candida has created a state of autoimmunity where the body's immune system seems to be attacking itself. Among related conditions Dr. Saifer includes hypothyroidism, thyroiditis, hypodadrenalism, Addison's disease, hepatitis, premenstrual syndrome, and rheumatoid arthritis. Although the mechanism is not clearly understood, these conditions seem to be triggered by toxins associated with candidiasis or systemic yeast infections.

Suzie's story

Suzie was 24 when I first saw her. A committed vegetarian, at her age Suzie should have been in vibrant good health with bags of energy. Instead she was suffering from chronic and debilitating fatigue, sugar cravings, occasional depression, waking up often during the night, PMS, irregular and painful periods, constipation, intestinal pain and low blood pressure. Blood tests showed her to be short of iron and a stool test showed up some parasite and candida infection. At one point her periods stopped completely for eight months.

At that time I wasn't using the thyroid temperature test mentioned in chapter 10, nor had I heard of APICH, but it was clear that Suzie was suffering from hormonal disruption that involved her thyroid and adrenal function, as well as her pituitary gland (the master gland controlling the production of oestrogens and progesterone). Chronic low blood pressure, period pain and irregularity and a low iron count are often a symptom of low thyroid function.

I started Suzie on an anti-candida programme and recommended a wide range of vitamins, minerals and essential fatty acids along with a specific herbal anti-fungal based on caprylic acid. I also recommended a supplement containing dulse and l-tyrosine for thyroid function and her doctor prescribed medication to take care of the parasite. For her leaky gut and to improve digestion and absorption, I recommended she take some betaine hydrochloride (weak stomach acid), digestive enzymes, probiotics (good intestinal bacteria) and a product containing l-glutamine to heal the intestinal membrane.

Suzie took a long time to start feeling the benefit of the nutritional programme, and often found it difficult keeping to it. She occasionally rang or emailed me in despair because she seemed to be taking three steps forward and then two back – feeling a bit better for a few days, then back to feeling unwell again. After five months her doctor told her she didn't have candida any more and she stopped her anti-candida programme. Within a couple of weeks all her symptoms had come back. She quickly realised the progress she had in fact already made and went straight back on the programme.

Later Suzie moved to another continent and about one year after first starting her programme I received an email telling me she felt absolutely marvellous. She was so happy she had decided to stick with the regime, even though it didn't seem to be working at first. She had no more period problems, her energy levels were high, and she was sleeping really well.

Suzie's recovery took a long time, but the endocrine system can be slow to get back in balance when it has been so badly disrupted.

Diagnosis of candidiasis syndrome

Candidiasis is a syndrome that goes largely unrecognised by the medical profession and is not generally acknowledged by the majority of doctors as an existing condition. I have found that when my clients have presented their doctor with the wide variety of symptoms that are associated with candidiasis (ranging from abdominal bloating/pain and constipation, lethargy and extreme fatigue, PMS and joint pains), the doctor is at a loss. Each symptom is treated individually and they are referred to gynaecologists, gastroenterologists and other specialists. When the symptoms don't respond to treatment, the patient despairs of finding a solution to their health problems.

Even when a medical practitioner is open to the possibility of candidiasis, it is hard to diagnose because everyone has candida present in their stools. A blood test can show IgE antibodies to candida and a stool test may show up pathological levels of candida, i.e. higher than expected amounts. However, not everyone with candidiasis makes antibodies to candida, and not everyone suffers from digestive problems yet they can still have fungal infections.

52

The candidiasis check list as a tool for diagnosis

The check list below gives a fair idea of whether or not you are suffering from candidiasis, although it is not always clear immediately as some people can be relatively well and still have candidiasis, while others feel terrible but are suffering from a 'simple' food intolerance or blood sugar problems. In the end, the assessment is made taking into account medical history and current health problems. Unless the symptoms are very severe or obviously pointing to a candidiasis problem, I prefer to assume other causes first and deal with the underlying blood sugar, leaky gut, digestive problems or hormonal imbalances. Often the candidiasis is brought naturally under control by the body's own defenses. If there are no improvements after the first month, then I resort to an anti-candida programme. Use the check list to see whether or not Candida is undermining your hormone health.

Candidiasis check list.
(Please highlight all symptoms)

Part One

In women:
- Persistent or recurrent cystitis, vaginitis, urethritis?
- Pelvic inflammatory disease or endometriosis?
- Thrush (oral or vaginal yeast infection) more than once a year?
- Premenstrual syndrome, period pain or irregularity, infertility?
- Vaginal discharge or irritation?
- Have you ever taken contraceptive medication (the Pill) or hormone replacement therapy (HRT) for a year or more?

In men:
- Prostate problems, infertility, impotence or loss of sex drive?
- Irritation or fungal infections around groin or genitals?

General:
- Urinary urgency, frequency or burning?
- Fungal infections of the hands, feet, nails or skin?
- Symptoms usually worse on damp days or in mouldy places?
- Have you taken antibiotics for longer than a month or more than once in a year?
- Have had a course of steroid treatment such as prednisolone, cortisone or ACTH, or been treated with immuno-suppressive drugs, e.g. after transplant surgery?

Part Two. Score symptoms:

Mild/occasional = 1. Frequent or moderately severe = 2. Severe or disabling = 3.

- Loss of sex drive?
- Allergies (food, chemical, dust mite, pollen etc)?
- Sensitivity to chemical smells, petrol fumes, perfumes, tobacco smoke?
- A draining fatigue not relieved by sleep, lethargy, poor memory, feelings of 'unreality' or 'spaciness'?
- Unaccountable muscle aches, tingling, numbness or burning?
- Unaccountable aches and swelling in joints?
- Headaches, migraines?
- Loss of balance, dizziness or lack of coordination?
- Depression, irritability, anxiety, mood swings, aggressive outbursts, loss of emotional equilibrium?
- Erratic vision or spots before the eyes?
- Eczema, psoriasis, skin rashes, itching?
- Dry mouth or throat, post-nasal drip, nasal itch and/or congestion, sinusitis?
- Tightness in chest, wheezing or shortness of breath?
- Sore throat, irritable cough, sores in mouth?
- Ear sensitivity or fluid in ears, recurrent ear infections, earache, deafness?
- Cravings for sweet foods, bread or alcohol?
- Persistent drowsiness, need for excessive sleep?
- Abdominal bloating, distension, diarrhoea or constipation, mucous in stools, irritable bowel syndrome?
- Heartburn, indigestion, belching, flatulence, anal irritation or itching?
- Bad breath, body odour?
- Have you ever had a high alcohol intake or taken recreational drugs?
- Have you ever had a high sugar diet, now or in the past (even as a child), or been through a very stressful period in your life?

How to score the checklist

Part one

If you have ticked one or more of the boxes in part one, this indicates that candidiasis is highly likely to be the cause of your health problems.

Part two

0 – 30:   You may have some candidiasis activity, but your symptoms
          may also be due to other causes
30 – 64: You appear to have some candida activity which is the
          probable cause of your symptoms
65 – 100 : Candida is highly indicated as the underlying cause of your
          symptoms and the reason you feel unwell

Candida and hormone balance

Because of its affinity with hormones, candida can have a profound effect on the endocrine system. It's a bit like throwing a spanner in the works. Candida disrupts one set of hormones, and the rest are thrown out of balance. The only time most women know they have candida is when they get a vaginal yeast infection (thrush). However, you can have candidiasis and not suffer from thrush. This means that many cases of candidiasis go undetected if thrush is not one of the symptoms present. Candidiasis can be an underlying cause of all sorts of hormonal disturbance.

Endometriosis

Endometriosis is a condition where the lining of the uterus (endometrium) grows outside the uterus in other parts of the abdominal cavity. It can (rarely) migrate to other parts of the body and has even been found around the heart. When the uterus lining is shed and bleeds once a month, so does the endometrial tissue; wherever it has transplanted itself. Symptoms can vary from mild to very severe. Some women can have it and not be aware until they have an ultra sound examination. For others, like Kim (story below), the endometriosis can be rampant, affecting a woman's whole health.

According to Kristi New Myer, MD in her informative website, endometriosis was first described by Daniel Shroen in 1690 in Disputatio Inauguralis Medica de Ulceribus Ulceri, in which he described sores throughout the "*stomach, bladder, intestines, and broad ligament which had a tendency to form adhesions that linked visceral areas together.*" Endometriosis is not a new disease.[52]

There is no consensus as to the cause(s) of endometriosis, but candidiasis is usually found to be a contributing factor to the progression of the disease, and along with PCBs (chapter 2), may even be the one factor that predisposes a woman to endometriosis. In 1996 the U.S. Endometriosis Association described the relationship of candida albicans and endometriosis in their newsletter, *"No other approach to endometriosis has given as consistent, long-term, positive results as the treatment for Candida albicans/allergy/infection and its related problems."*[53]

As endometriosis may also be due to an imbalance in oestrogen and progesterone, with oestrogen dominating, many of my clients with endometriosis who combine anti-candida therapy with natural progesterone derive great relief from their symptoms, without the risk of increased rates of cancer normally associated with conventional hormone treatment.

Kim's story

Kim started experiencing abdominal pains and cramps when she was 26, ten years previously. In the intervening years her symptoms had grown worse and eventually she was diagnosed as having endometriosis that had spread throughout her abdominal cavity, including her urethra and bladder.

She had several operations, including one to remove a very large cyst growing on her ovary. Each time she saw a specialist, she was told she had to take the Pill as this was the only way she would keep the endometriosis from spreading. However, Kim's intuition told her that in her case, taking the synthetic hormones was only making things worse. She had originally started taking the Pill when she was 17 for her period pains, and was convinced that this had been at least partly responsible for her condition.

When she came to see me, Kim had spent a lot of time researching endometriosis on the internet and discovered that indeed, in some women, taking the Pill can 'feed' this disease. She stopped taking the hormones straight away. Kim had also discovered the connection between endometriosis and candidiasis. However, the response from the various specialists she talked to was very discouraging. She couldn't find anyone who acknowledged the existence of candidiasis, let alone that it might be undermining her chances of recovery. Kim was feeling very low. She had recently had more tests done and her doctor thought her endometriosis may have spread to inside her intestines.

Kim's other symptoms confirmed that she was on the right track when she suspected a candida infection. As well as endometriosis, Kim also suffered from asthma and an allergic reaction to dust mite, grass, cats, dogs and pollen, chronic fatigue, morning headaches, fungal infections on her toe nails, vaginal thrush, gallstones, constipation, haemorrhoids, indigestion, abdominal bloating and poor blood sugar control - all associated with candida infection when so many symptoms occur at once. No matter what she ate, Kim felt uncomfortable as though she couldn't process her food any more and the constipation was making her feel miserable.

I started Kim on an anti-candida, hypoallergenic programme that included supplements for healing the intestinal membrane, to help with digestion, absorption and elimination, and to directly kill off the candida infection.

She also took a wide range of vitamins, minerals and essential fatty acids to help her body start the healing process. In addition, I recommended natural progesterone cream for its ability to reduce oestrogen dominance. Then Kim was recommended a nutritionally orientated doctor who specialised in endocrine dysfunction. He encouraged her to stick with the nutrition programme and gave a big 'yes' to the natural progesterone cream.

When I saw her two months later, Kim was feeling a million times better. In her words, "Two to three weeks after coming to see you, I woke up one morning and thought, this is how I am supposed to feel." Kim had rediscovered her natural energy levels. It was very early days, but Kim found she had no more problems with digesting food and the constipation was slowly getting better, her period pain had stopped and more important, an ultra sound examination showed that her endometriosis was under control.

Six months later, Kim was the picture of radiant health and vitality. She still followed the programme faithfully and continued with her supplements and the natural progesterone cream. I had explained that it could take a good year to reverse all her long standing health problems. With her enlightened doctor to monitor her progress, Kim felt well taken care of and knew intuitively that she was creating good health, not just masking her symptoms.

Chronic and interstitial cystitis (IC)

Interstitial cystitis is a condition resulting in recurring discomfort or pain in the bladder and the surrounding pelvic region. The symptoms of IC vary from case to case and even in the same individual. People may experience mild discomfort, pressure, tenderness, or intense pain in the bladder and surrounding pelvic area. Symptoms may include an urgent need to urinate, frequent need to urinate, or a combination of these symptoms. Pain may change in intensity as the bladder fills with urine or as it empties. Women's symptoms often get worse during menstruation.

In IC, the bladder wall is irritated and becomes scarred or stiff. Glomerulations (pinpoint bleeding caused by recurrent irritation) may appear. Some people with IC find that their bladders cannot hold much urine, which increases the frequency of urination, despite having a normal bladder capacity. People with severe cases of IC may urinate as many as 60 times a day and they often experience pain during sexual intercourse. While men can also have IC, 90% of sufferers are women.[54]

Angie's story

When Angie first came to see me she was taking regular medication for IC from which she had been suffering for about 18 months. She had been told there was no cure and she would need to take the medication (Elmiron) probably for ever. Just prior to her IC symptoms starting, Angie had been treated for poison ivy with steroid injections, including prednisolone. The steroids caused eczema and a severe bout of vaginal thrush. The IC started soon after, with pain particularly during intercourse. More lately she had been feeling permanently tired, had frequent headaches, depression, stomach pains and diarrhoea. Since a radical hysterectomy 10 years previously, Angie had been taking hormone replacement. Provera (progestogens) had caused side effects, so she was taking unopposed oestrogen in the form of Premarin. She also used Canderel, a sweetener containing aspartame.

Chronic cystitis and thrush are symptoms that strongly indicate a candida infection. The steroid treatment she received for the poison ivy had been the most likely trigger for candidiasis, destroying good intestinal bacteria and allowing candida to flourish. I was concerned that Angie was taking unopposed oestrogen as candida loves extra circulating hormones and unopposed oestrogen increases the risk for cancer. According to the National Kidney and Urologic Diseases Information Clearinghouse

58

website, some research has also pointed to the use of aspartame as a bladder irritant.

I suggested that Angie start an anti-candida nutrition programme, avoiding all sugar, yeast, dairy foods, refined carbohydrates and fermented foods such as alcohol and vinegar. She also had to avoid nutritional stressors such as coffee, tea and chocolate. I recommended a range of supplements that included herbal anti-fungals, such as pau d'arco and garlic, along with vitamins, minerals and essential fatty acids.

Two months later Angie had had no reoccurrence of her thrush which was unusual for her because she had been swimming a lot and that normally brought it on. Neither had she experienced any more cystitis, despite stopping her medication. She also felt less tired.

Five months later, Angie had stopped the Premarin and given up her last one Canderel per day. She suffered no more headaches, diarrhoea or stomach pains and had had no cystitis since starting the programme, even when she came off the Elmiron.

CHAPTER 7
ALLERGIES AND FOOD INTOLERANCE

What is allergy?

Certain conditions are known as 'classical allergic disorders', and include hayfever, asthma, perennial rhinitis, urticaria and eczema. These conditions are recognised by the mainstream medical profession because they give a positive result on a skin prick test. This test involves inserting, either by scratching or pricking, a purified extract of the suspected allergen under the skin and waiting for a localised inflammatory response.

Raised levels of IgE (immunoglobulin E) in the blood also help with positive diagnosis of classical allergy. IgE is one of the five classes of antibodies known as immunoglobulins (round protein molecules involved with immunity). On exposure to an antigen, IgE antibodies attach themselves to the surface of the mast cells of the immune system which are stimulated to release histamine, plus other chemical messengers, to alert the rest of the immune system. Histamine causes the inflammatory response associated with allergic reaction. In cases of allergy, the mast cells are being stimulated to produce excessive amounts of histamine. Allergy is a form of over-reaction to an inappropriate stimulus.

Intolerance/sensitivity

Since the 1980's, thanks to allergy specialists like Dr. Jonathan Brostoff, masked (or delayed) allergies are becoming much more widely accepted even though the concept does not conform to the mainstream view of allergy.[55] These are responses which can take hours or even days to materialise and cannot immediately be related to foods commonly eaten, or substances with which the sufferer is constantly in contact. They also do not necessarily show up on an orthodox allergy test. In fact you can have an altered reaction to almost any food or chemical substance, without it necessarily being measurable.

Intolerance can provoke a wide variety of symptoms, most of which are not life threatening, but can have debilitating effects on health, including skin problems, ear, nose and throat disorders (including sinusitis), digestive upsets (including IBS), aching muscles and joints, loss of memory, concentration and coordination, mood swings, irritability and depression, water retention, vaginal discharge and sensitivity to other substances such as pollen, animal fur, house dust mite, car fumes, cigarette smoke, perfume, etc.

How food intolerance develops

People can be born with allergies, usually inheriting them from parents, in which case the sensitivities are passed from one generation to the next. Allergies can also develop as a result of damage to the intestinal membrane (leaky gut). Sometimes it's a combination of inherited reaction and leaky gut. An elimination diet based on stone age principles can bring a relief to symptoms, even when the allergy is to an outside agent, such as house dust mite or pollen and is an inherited condition.

Stone age inheritance

In his book, *"Stone Age Diet. The Natural Way to Eat"*,[56] Leon Chaitow talks about maladaptation to certain food groups as a cause of many allergy-related health problems. Researchers looked at what human beings ate when they were hunter gatherers, before they settled and started farming around 10,000 years ago. They discovered that our hunter gatherer ancestors consumed very few of their calories in the form of grains (cereals) and dairy produce. Nor did they consume simple sugars (white sugar). Grains and dairy produce figured much more prominently in our diets when neolithic man started growing grains and keeping animals. Some researchers argue that, genetically speaking, our physical evolution is still at the stone age stage and that many of us are less well adapted to the consumption of grains and dairy produce than are others – modern 'stone-agers'. Stone-agers also have less tolerance to other more modern foods like sugar, coffee, tea, alcohol, and processed foods.

Allergy and hormones

While not usually thought of as being connected to hormone problems, sensitivity or intolerance to anything you are eating can cause reactive hypoglycaemia. Reactive hypoglycaemia means a sudden drop in blood sugar in response to certain foods. As blood sugar control and hormone stability are closely linked, this can have an effect on your symptoms.

Food intolerances also cause metabolic disturbances that can affect your endocrine system directly, as well as reducing energy and making you tired. Many women report a rise in energy levels, a clearing of their brain 'fog' and a reduction in PMS symptoms when they avoid foods to which they are sensitive.

Leaky gut

People who suffer from any kind of allergy or sensitivity to foods, drinks or outside agents usually have a leaky gut. They may also have candidiasis, but leaky gut can exist without the presence of candida infection.

Asthma, eczema and hayfever sufferers usually have a wide range of food intolerances, despite being told that their allergy is due solely to an environmental agent. Once the offending food substances are removed from the diet, and the leaky gut is allowed to heal, environmental allergies usually go away. I have known numbers of women who suffered from hayfever, eczema and asthma find their symptoms just disappeared when they followed an elimination diet and took supplements to heal a leaky gut.

Common food culprits

You can become sensitive or intolerant to almost anything, but the most common foods to cause a reaction are:

- All gluten-containing grains, especially wheat, but also oats, rye and barley
- All grains, including gluten-free grains (rice, buckwheat, maize and millet)
- Milk products (milk, cheese, yoghurt, cream, sour cream, cottage cheese and ice cream) - whether from cows, sheep or goats
- Eggs
- Soya (soya milk, soya yoghurt, soya cheese, miso, soy sauce, tofu, tempeh and tamari)
- Citrus fruits
- Nightshade family (potatoes, aubergines, bell peppers and tomatoes)
- Nuts, especially peanuts (not strictly a nut but a legume as peanuts grow underground)
- Sugar, chocolate, coffee, tea, alcohol and tobacco

Elimination diets

Apart from medical testing involving skin prick tests or blood tests to pick up an immune response to allergens, the most reliable way of discovering food sensitivities is to follow an elimination diet, avoiding the most common foods known to be involved in allergic response, for up to one month. Then use the allergy pulse test to see which foods are safe to re-introduce into the diet.

Allergy pulse test

The allergy pulse test is based on the principle that when you avoid suspected foods for a period of time (a minimum of 14 days – 28 days is better), and then re-introduce the food in a controlled challenge, the body will go into first stage reaction, or alarm state, and cause an appreciable rise in blood pressure and exaggerated symptoms.

Avoid the substances you are testing strictly for 14 days. I suggest you start with the most common food allergens: wheat, milk products, soya and eggs. I am assuming that if you have hormone disruption that you have already dropped coffee, tea, sugar and alcohol from your diet!

After 14 days of complete abstinence you take an hour when you feel calm and will have no interruptions. Record your resting pulse rate then eat a larger than normal portion of the food you are testing, for example a large chunk of bread (for wheat and yeast) or a large bowl of pasta (for wheat alone). Over the course of the next hour record your pulse rate after 10 minutes, half an hour and one hour later. Over the next 24 hours, record any symptoms you might experience. If you have a rise in pulse rate as well as symptoms, that is a good indication that you have sensitivity to that food. You should wait 48 hours before testing the next food. No reaction means you can test the next food after 24 hours.

One woman told me how she suspected she was sensitive to the nightshade family and did her allergy pulse test on potatoes. Within an hour of eating potatoes she was so overcome with fatigue that she had to go to bed for the afternoon! She had been feeling fine before the challenge. A couple of others both reported feeling quite ill and wobbly for at least 24 hours after challenging with cheese and wheat. The more violent the reaction, the more harm those foods were doing you while you were eating them.

If you have a reaction, you will certainly have to continue avoiding that substance for three months, about the length of time it takes to heal a leaky gut. After that time, you may well be able to consume the offending food on a 'rotational' basis, i.e. eating it only every three days to allow it time to be cleared from your system till the next time of eating. This avoids a build up of reaction and a return to chronic sensitivity.

Advantages of the allergy pulse test

The beauty of the allergy pulse test is that you can re-test foods periodically to see if you are still sensitive to them. It also allows you to track any changing sensitivities which can occur as a result of religiously substituting one food for another. For example, people who use soya milk consistently in place of cow's milk, without dealing with the underlying causes of the sensitivity, can develop an intolerance to soya products too.

I have used the allergy pulse test successfully for some years now. It is non invasive, simple and can be done by individuals themselves in their own homes. It gives a good idea which foods you are sensitive to at this moment in your life. As food intolerance can be a changing phenomenon, it is important to discover what you should avoid at this moment in your health recovery programme.

CHAPTER 8
LOW THYROID FUNCTION

The thyroid is a butterfly-shaped gland situated in the neck (diagram 1, chapter 3). It is the largest endocrine gland in the body and secretes thyroid hormones that regulate metabolism, i.e. the rate at which the body 'burns fuel' to create energy. Thyroid hormones also control the rate of protein synthesis required for growth, maintenance and repair of the body, and for normal maturation of the nervous system. With low thyroid function (hypothyroidism), body temperature drops as the rate for fuel burning decreases. This leads to a reduction in heat production. At the same time, growth and body repair slow down or stop, while water, salts and protein are retained and blood cholesterol goes up.[57]

Thyroid function is initiated by the hypothalamus and controlled by the pituitary gland, both known as the 'master glands' because they exert control over the adrenals, ovaries and testes, as well as the thyroid. The pituitary releases thyroid stimulating hormone (TSH) which stimulates the thyroid to secrete thyroxine (T4) and triiodothyronine (T3), known collectively as thyroid hormone (TH). Iodine is essential for the production of TH.

In her article, "Underactive thyroid. A nutritional approach" appearing in the Summer Edition 2002 of the Optimum Nutrition Journal, Karen Goodfellow, BSc, Bed(Hons) DPSN, Research Officer for Thyroid UK explains that approximately 80% of the hormone secreted by the thyroid is T4. This must then be converted in the liver and muscles to T3, the active form of thyroid hormone, using an enzyme called deiodinase. Production of T3 is designed to meet energy demand. As activity increases, so does the production of T3. When low thyroid function exists, T3 does not keep up with energy demand resulting in exhaustion and the many symptoms associated with hypothyroidism.[58]

Hypothyroidism check list

The thyroid check list shows the many functions that are influenced by the thyroid. Take a look to see whether or not your hormone problems are linked to low thyroid function.

Weight, appetite and water retention

- Inability to lose weight despite following a sensible weight loss programme
- Poor or loss of appetite with no weight loss, or even weight gain
- Inexplicable weight loss (should always be medically investigated)
- Chronic water retention, including swelling of face, only relieved by strong anti-diuretics

Skin, nails, hair, tongue and voice

- Hair loss not related to male pattern baldness, loss of hair on lower third of legs, scanty eyebrows
- Skin problems such as acne, eczema or psoriasis, rough, dry, flaky or 'papery' skin, orange peel appearance or lemon tinge to skin
- Reddish tinge to cheeks each side of the nose
- Swollen tongue with scalloped edge
- Nails grow slowly, tend to be weak, brittle and ridged (ridges going both ways)
- Hoarse voice
- Pallor (growing pale)

Sleep, energy and fatigue

- Fatigue, lack of energy and exhaustion not relieved by rest or sleep
- Insomnia, sleep apnoea and snoring
- Chronic fatigue syndrome / ME

Temperature control

- Constantly feel cold, even in a warm environment, hands, feet, extremities always cold
- Heat intolerance

Digestive, liver and kidney problems

- Chronic constipation only temporarily relieved by fibre or laxatives
- Abdominal bloating, flatulence, indigestion, heartburn, nausea, anal irritation or itching
- Gallstones, abnormal liver enzymes (elevated AST and ALT)
- Reduced kidney filtration, kidney stones

Aches and pains

- Frequent and often debilitating headaches or migraines
- Unaccounted for muscle and joint pains or stiffness, particularly worse in the morning, after sitting or on damp days
- Numbness in the limbs, "pins and needles", especially in the hands upon waking
- Fybromyalgia[59]

Sexual and reproductive dysfunction

- Loss of sex drive, impotence, infertility, miscarriage
- Menstruation difficulties, e.g. heavy painful periods, irregular periods or loss of periods

Cardiovascular health

- High cholesterol, high blood fats, high or low blood pressure
- Heart murmurs, palpitations
- Chronic iron deficiency anaemia that returns when iron supplements are discontinued

Eyes and ears

- Night blindness
- Deafness particularly in right ear, tinnitus

Immunity

- Frequent infections
- Multiple allergies

Blood sugar and mental health

- Poor memory and inability to concentrate, increased irritability, mental dullness, depression
- Blood sugar problems, e.g. hypo- or hyper-glycaemia, diabetes

Adapted from "Hypothyroidism: The Unsuspected Illness" by Broda O. Barnes MD and Lawrence Galton, and "Solved: The Riddle of Illness – Your Amazing Thyroid ...", by Dr. Stephen E. Langer[60]

Factors that upset the thyroid gland

Stress, as well as many environmental and nutritional factors can affect the thyroid.

Exposure to radiation

Chernobyl affected many people who were exposed to the fall out. Exposure to radiation can also come from x-rays and radon, which is naturally present in ground rock in some geographical locations such as the south west of England (Cornwall) and the Channel Islands (Jersey). People living in close proximity to a nuclear power reactor may be affected by radiation.

Lack of nutrients

Iodine, selenium and zinc are required for the activation of TH (thyroid hormone). Vitamin A, the B vitamins, zinc and the amino acid tyrosine also play an important part in thyroid health.

Some foods

Members of the cabbage family (brussels sprouts, turnips, cauliflower, cabbage and kale) contain glucosinolates, known as a goitrogenic chemical as they interfere with the thyroid gland causing it to swell (known as a goitre). This effect only occurs in the presence of iodine deficiency and is reduced if these vegetables are cooked.

Soya beans contain the compounds diadzein and genistein (isoflavones) that may block thyroid peroxidase (TPO), an enzyme required for the synthesis of TH. Daniel R. Doerge, Ph.D., a researcher at the Food and Drug Administration's National Center for Toxicological Research, has researched soya's anti-thyroid properties, and advises against soy supplements or eating huge amounts of soya foods because *"there is definitely potential for interaction with the thyroid."*[61] However, not all research is that cut and dried, and other studies show the opposite, that small amounts of soya can actually increase thyroid activity.[62,63]

Soya beans are not the only food that contain TPO inhibitors. Millet contains high levels of flavinoids, and can be problematic for thyroid function.[63]

However, this should not deter women from consuming fermented soya products such as miso, tempeh and tamari, plus small amounts of tofu, if liked. This is the way soya is consumed in Asian countries where incidence of hormone-related cancers is low. Isoflavones have been found to be the protective factor in fermented soya foods, because they help balance hormones naturally by blocking out the effect of environmental oestrogens (chapter 2). This is not the same as drinking soya milk, which is not fermented and currently not highly recommended (chapter 11).

Environmental toxins

Fluoride and chlorides both block the uptake of iodine by the thyroid (chapter 10). Avoid fluoride in toothpastes and mouth washes and filter tap water to filter out fluorides.

PCBs (polychlorinated biphenyls) alter the structure of the thyroid gland, inhibiting its ability to respond to hormone signals. PCBs also increase the excretion of T4 and they block the entry of thyroid hormone into cells.[65,66]

Mercury

Amalgam or silver fillings contain mercury which blocks T4 production and its conversion to T3 by interfering with selenium and zinc metabolism – both of which are required for TH production.

Medications

A long list of medications can interfere with thyroid function and includes steroids, beta blockers, insulin, diazepam and lithium, some tranquilisers, salicylates (found in aspirin and dispirin), anti-convulsants, levodopa and bromocriptine (for treating Parkinson's disease), antacids, cholesterol lowering drugs, tamoxifen and hormones found in HRT and the Pill. For more detailed information, check out the Thyroid UK website.[67]

Oestrogen

Oestrogen reduces the amount of available thyroid hormone while raising overall levels. This gives the impression of having adequate thyroid hormone when in fact less is available for use by receptor cells. If you are taking any kind of oestrogen medication, make sure you have your TSH levels checked periodically to to see if the oestrogen is having an effect on thyroid function.

Stress

Stress works via the hypothalamus which has a direct effect on all of the endocrine system, including thyroid function.[68] But whether or not the thyroid is affected by stress varies from one person to another, the same as with any health problems. A well nourished thyroid that hasn't been exposed to too many anti-thyroid agents should not be affected in the long term by stress.

Diagnosing hypothyroidism

My experience with women who have many symptoms associated with low thyroid function is that when they go for a blood test, the results very often come back as normal. This is very puzzling until you realise that what doctors normally check for is levels of T4, on the assumption that providing there is sufficient T4, it will be converted to T3, the active form or thyroid hormone. However, T4 doesn't always get converted to T3 if the conditions are not favourable for T4 to T3 conversion. A deficiency in selenium will affect T4 to T3 conversion.

The Barnes basal temperature test, described below, gives a more accurate picture of thyroid health. It's dead easy to do and, like the allergy pulse test, it is non-invasive, costs nothing and can be done simply in the privacy of your own home. If you find your basal temperature is below the normal range over a couple of tests, then do go back to your doctor and ask for more sensitive thyroid function testing. Remember that taking medication may be affecting your thyroid function and taking oestrogen may give a false impression of adequate thyroid hormone.

The Barnes basal temperature test

Because of temperature fluctuations during the monthly cycle (it is highest shortly before the start of the menstrual flow and lowest at the time of ovulation), a woman in her menstruating years should take her temperature on the second and third days of her period after the flow has started. Girls who haven't started their periods, postmenopausal women and men can take their temperature on any day of the week.

Take a thermometer to bed with you. Shake it down well and place on the bedside table. Immediately upon waking in the morning, place the thermometer snugly in the armpit for ten minutes. A reading below the normal range of 97.8°F to 98.2°F or 36°C to 37.2°C strongly suggests low thyroid function. If the reading is above the normal range, it is an indication of an infection or an overactive thyroid gland.

Medical treatment for low thyroid function

Current medical treatment for low thyroid function are the synthetic hormones, Levothyroxine, Eltroxin and Liothyronine. However, I have seen many women who are taking thyroid medication and yet still have all the symptoms associated with low thyroid function. According to Dr. Stephen Langer, synthetic thyroid medications provide plenty of T4 on the assumption that the body will convert this to T3. But this does not always work well in practice. He and many doctors in both the U.S. and Europe are going against conventional medical wisdom and using natural thyroid extract, such as Armour Thyroid (extracted from pig thyroid). Armour contains the full complement of thyroid hormones, including T3.[69,70,71]

Healthy thyroid, naturally

The thyroid responds to nutritional support - just like the rest of the body - and whatever you do to support your health through optimum nutrition will have a beneficial effect on the whole of the endocrine system. There are specific supplements available for thyroid support based on seaweed for iodine and other minerals, the amino acids l-glutamine, l-glycine and l-tyrosine, zinc, selenium, the B vitamins and vitamins A and E. Because they are so effective, I make sure that anyone already taking prescribed thyroid medication has their dose regularly checked as it often needs to be reduced. Symptoms of too much thyroid medication are heart palpitations, sweating, feeling jittery and agitated, muscle cramping, headache, restlessness, flushing and diarrhoea.

Important!

Whatever you do, do not stop prescribed thyroid medication. If you have any doubts about your medication, you must discuss it with your prescribing medical practitioner.

Now let's take a look at the next stage in a woman's life.

CHAPTER 9
THE MENOPAUSE

Often referred to as 'the change', menopause literally means the end of periods, but is most commonly used to describe the gradual process during which a woman stops menstruating. The changes can start to take place any time from 40 onwards and in most women menopause is completed by around 55. There are exceptions. I know of one or two women who are still menstruating regularly every month at age 56. Period regularity is usually the first change that women notice. Periods may suddenly become unpredictable, irregular and lighter, or less often but heavier. All these variations can go on for between four and six years as oestrogen and progesterone levels start to decline.

At the menopause a woman's ovaries still produce some oestrogen, although in smaller quantities and not enough to prepare her uterus for pregnancy, for at least twelve years after the start of the menopause. Progesterone levels fall dramatically and eventually their production in the ovaries stops altogether.[72]

Menopause is brought about by the using up of all the eggs in a woman's ovaries. Usually by the age of 45 a women has fewer egg follicles and oestrogen levels have started to decrease. Irregular periods at this time are usually anovulatory, meaning that while she continues to have periods, a woman does not ovulate as often due to the decreasing supply of eggs. It can therefore be more difficult for women in their 40's to conceive (though don't assume you won't!). Lack of ovulation naturally causes a drop in progesterone production as progesterone is only produced in the ovaries following the release of a mature egg.

There are three main phases to the menopause:

Perimenopause

Menstruation still occurs but hormone shifts have begun and changes in regularity of periods, the heaviness of flow and the length of time will have started. This can happen anywhere between the ages of 40 and 50. Periods will start being anovulatory.

Some symptoms may be experienced with the drop in both oestrogen and progesterone levels. Most common symptoms include hot flushes, sleeplessness, night sweats, mood swings, weight gain, loss of sex drive. The degree to which women are affected varies from one individual to another.

Menopause

This is the time when the last period occurs, although you will not know it was your last period until you reach the next stage 12 – 18 months later! Some women can go six months without a period and then another one arrives. The end of the reproductive years rarely coincides with the last period. Fertility can have finished before then due to anovulatory periods or it can continue up to 18 months after the last period. For this reason it is important to continue using some form of contraception if you really don't want to get pregnant again.

Postmenopause

You know you are in this phase when you have not had a period for at least 12 months, and certainly after 18 months of no periods. But you have not been left bereft of hormones. Your ovaries still continue for a few more years producing small amounts of oestrogen, while both oestrogen and progesterone continue to be produced in the adrenals, liver, fat cells and muscles. How effectively the adrenals will continue this role depends on the amount of stress from nutritional stressors, poor diet, nutritional deficiencies and unhealthy lifestyle to which they have been exposed in their lifetime. Healthy adrenals will continue to produce these hormones for life, and will help to relieve the change over period as the ovaries start to shut down. They also produce androgens (male hormones), including testosterone, which can give postmenopausal women renewed energy and zest for life, as well as helping maintain libido.[73] Your reproductive years may have come to an end, but life after the ups and downs of monthly cycles is just beginning!

Testing for the menopause

Because of lower levels of oestrogen and progesterone, FSH and LH levels go unchecked and start to rise. If a blood test shows rising levels of FSH and LH, it means you are likely to be menopausal.

Table 1 is a typical blood test result (mine!) of a perimenopausal woman, showing the normal reference ranges for menstruating women for comparison.

Phase	FSH MUI/ml	LH MUI/ml	Oestradiol Pg/ml	Progesterone Ng/ml
Patient's Results	54.4	48.7	10	0.4
Reference ranges for comparison				
Follicular (1st half of the month)	2.5 - 10.2	1.9 - 12.5	11 - 165	0.2 – 1.4
Ovulatory	3.4 – 33.4	8.7 – 76.3	146 – 526	-
Luteal (2nd half of the month)	1,5 – 9.2	0.5 – 16.9	33 – 196	3.3 - 28
Menopausal	23 – 116.3	15.9 – 54	< 37	< 0.7

Table 1. Blood test result for peri-menopausal woman

If you have had blood test results and compare them with the above, you may find the reference ranges quoted on your results slightly different to the ones here. This is because there can be variations in the reference ranges used from one laboratory to another.

Fat or thin?

Because body fat is a manufacturing plant for oestrogen, low or no fat diets are a big mistake for women. Don't be tempted to lose too much weight by following a fat-free diet. It is natural to put on a little weight during the 40s and battling to relive your weight at age 20 (providing you were thin then!) usually ends in frustration and a feeling of failure. Better to do regular exercise and have a toned, fit and shapely body than to be thin and bony as you enter the menopause.

However, it is not an excuse to put on excessive amounts of weight either! Fat cells store environmental oestrogens as well as making their own, and an imbalance can lead to oestrogen dominance and an increased risk for breast cancer.

Following a diet containing essential fatty acids that help your hormones function correctly is preferable to following a no- or low- fat diet (chapter 12). Low fat diets don't differentiate among the different types of fats. Low fat prepared meals, designed for weight conscious people, just contain lower amounts of the same type of fat, i.e. high in harmful trans fatty acids. The shortfall in taste due to the reduced fat content is often made up with sugar or other refined carbohydrates. If you are too busy or too tired to prepare meals from scratch, try making an omelette, opening a can of tuna or slicing open an avocado and eating with a mixed salad and a cold pressed oil dressing. If you do need to buy a prepared meal from time to time, make sure you add a pile of raw or lightly cooked vegetables to eat with it and use a cold pressed oil salad dressing drizzled on the vegetables (chapter 17 for meal ideas).

Essential fatty acids are found in all seeds and nuts, and in the cold pressed oils made from them. In your local health food shop and some well stocked supermarkets, you are likely to have a choice among linseed, sunflower, safflower, olive, corn, sesame, pumpkin seed, hazelnut and walnut oils. Buy organic where you can. Except for olive and peanut oil (which solidify in the cold), keep all cold pressed oils in the fridge and use them up quickly.

Symptoms associated with the menopause

Anecdotal reports of the symptoms associated with going through the menopause are enough to frighten most women into taking drastic action such as starting HRT (hormone replacement therapy). However, I have spoken to doctors who tell me that the vast majority of women sail through the menopause with only minor symptoms that are not enough to worry them. Some of it depends on attitude. If you regard the odd night sweat or hot flush as a natural indication of declining oestrogen and progesterone levels, it will not cause as much anxiety as someone who expects to feel exactly the same as they did before the changes started happening.

The women who do not sail through the menopause can experience severe, disrupting symptoms that can make their life hell. Here are the symptoms most commonly associated with changes in hormone levels. You may have some or all of them to a lesser or greater degree.

Physical symptoms

Hot flushes, dizziness, insomnia, night sweats, headaches, weight gain, water retention (bloating), vaginal itching, soreness and dryness, pain during intercourse, sore gums, joint pain, backache, muscle pain, hair loss, fatigue, loss of concentration, loss of memory, allergies, reduced immunity.

Emotional symptoms

Mood swings, irritability, depression, anxiety, panic attacks, loss of libido (sex drive).

Not a hormone deficiency disease

I have heard the menopause being likened to diabetes. The logic being that diabetes is a hormone deficiency disease (in this case insulin), and when the body does not produce enough, then it can be taken in the form of medication. The same argument goes for the menopause. As a woman becomes 'deficient' in oestrogen, she needs to replace it with medication, i.e. HRT. This is a false analogy because not every woman will get diabetes, but as sure as night follows day, every woman will go through the menopause, providing she lives long enough. It is a natural process and not a hormone deficiency disease. While menopausal symptoms are due to the reduction in oestrogen and progesterone production, with good nutritional support and a healthy lifestyle, the menopause should be a painless transition from menstruating to non-menstruating years. The changes take place over a number of years, making it a very gradual process.

Whatever your symptoms, you may well benefit from the nutritional advice in this book. Do seek medical advice as it is very important to have a thorough check up and diagnosis before assuming that your symptoms are due to the menopause.

Assessing the imbalances

The environmental and nutritional influences on hormones during the menopausal years are pretty much the same as during the menstruating years. The same kind of eating habits and the same supplements can help rebalance hormones. I base my assessment of menopausal problems on the same criteria I use for assessing menstrual problems. The following is my 10 point plan to check imbalances and the different influences on hormone health during the menopause. Each is covered in more detail in the chapters indicated.

Ten point hormone health analysis plan

1. **Digestion, absorption and elimination**

   This is the ability to digest and absorb nutrients, especially minerals such as calcium and magnesium, from food and eliminate toxins and hormones before they have a chance to get reactivated and reabsorbed (chapters 14).

2. **Blood sugar balance**

Symptoms of low blood sugar often correspond to symptoms associated with menopause, especially hot flushes, night sweats and fatigue (chapter 13).

3. **Low thyroid function**

The thyroid is an integral part of the endocrine system. Problems associated with low thyroid function can influence a women's menopause (chapter 8).

4. **Candidiasis and leaky gut**

A systemic yeast or fungal infection, candidiasis has an affinity with hormones and can have a profound effect on changing hormone balance as well as being a cause of vaginal soreness (chapter 6).

5. **Allergies and food intolerance**

Food intolerance drains energy, upsets blood sugar balance and can lead to exacerbated menopausal symptoms (chapter 7).

6. **Nutritional deficiencies**

Menopausal women benefit in the form of increased energy, sex drive, and emotional and mental stability when they redress vitamin, mineral and essential fatty acid deficiencies (chapter 15).

7. **Dietary habits**

Busy women tend to eat less than optimally balanced diets. Discovering short cuts to healthy eating and incorporating good habits into daily routine can make all the difference between feeling tired and out of balance and on top of the world, full of menopausal zest (chapter 11).

8. **Stress levels**

All forms of stress, whether emotional or environmental, can have a major influence on declining levels of hormones (chapter 1).

9. **Oestrogen/progesterone balance**

Usually requires a blood or saliva test for accurate assessment, however symptoms associated with oestrogen dominance give a good indication of the balance between oestrogen and progesterone (chapter 2).

10. Current medication, including HRT

What effects may medication be having on long term hormonal health? Are symptoms being experienced due to side effects of medication rather than the menopause itself?

Jane's story

Jane was in her late 40's and had started having hot flushes and night sweats. She had also been feeling tired, irritable and anxious since the birth of her second child eleven years previously. Keen on playing tennis, Jane was finding it hard to drag herself around the tennis court any more because her energy levels were so low.

I recommended some basic dietary changes for Jane that included cutting down on tea, coffee and sugary snacks, as these were affecting her blood sugar levels, and to include more fruit, vegetables, raw nuts and seeds. As she enjoyed cooking, Jane found the changes relatively easy to make. The supplements I recommended included a good multi vitamin and mineral with high levels of B vitamins (50 mg twice a day) and optimum amounts of zinc, selenium and iron. I also recommended vitamin E for the hot flushes, calcium and magnesium to help with her irritability and nervous tension, and a plant based supplement containing phytosterols to gently regulate hormone levels.

Just a month after starting the supplements and making the dietary modifications, Jane called me to say that she was feeling heaps better. Her hot flushes and night sweats had just about stopped and her energy levels had gone up so much she was now regularly beating her friends at tennis. She felt very optimistic about having a trouble-free menopause now she knew how to keep her hormones in balance.

Early menopause

Some women don't start having any signs of menopause until they are well into their fifties. Others start in their early forties. Geraldine, who came to one of my workshops, told me she had started an early menopause in her late thirties and was told by her doctor that she would need to start taking HRT. Determined not to have her menopause so early, Geraldine decided to change her eating habits, adding tofu and fermented soya products, cutting out alcohol, coffee, sugar and tea, and using linseeds and linseed oil. Within a couple of months her periods reappeared and continued to be regular well into her mid forties.

Stress or a shock can bring about an early menopause. I have talked to numbers of women who went through a very stressful period or had a shock in their late thirties or early forties and started an early menopause. Sometimes periods just stop overnight. For other women period irregularity and some symptoms of menopause, such as hot flushes and night sweats, start much earlier than expected due to prolonged periods of extreme stress. Stress affects the endocrine system via the hypothalamus and the pituitary glands. It can, therefore, have a profound effect on the ovaries, causing them to reduce their hormone output and bring on an earlier than expected menopause.

HRT – let's end the debate here

When I sent out some publicity about one of my menopause and osteoporosis workshops recently, I received a very strong reaction from Elise who thought I was being irresponsible for talking about statistics of 35%-50% increased cancer risk applying to women on HRT. She responded, *"If such statistics were true, then surely there would have been a huge outcry, especially as most doctors are prescribing HRT on demand or recommending it as soon as a woman starts peri-menopause"*.

My reply was to quote a small sample of the many studies that have been done on the dangers of HRT. The following are quoted from What Doctors Don't Tell You, *"HRT: the myths exploded" and "HRT: more bad news..."*[74]

A recent study of postmenopausal women found an astonishing 51% increased risk of breast cancer with 10 or more years of oestrogen-progesterone use, a risk level never reached with 15 years of using oestrogen alone *(J Natl Cancer Inst, 2000; 92:328-32)*

Data from a long term US Nurse's Health Study showed that the excess risk of cancer among those taking oestrogen alone was 32%, but 41% for those taking an oestrogen-progestogen combination. Overall, women taking hormones for five or more years had a 46% greater risk of breast cancer than those who were not. (N Engl J Med, 1995;332:1589-93).

The use of HRT increased the overall risk of invasive cancers with a "favourable prognosis" by nearly four and a half times. (JAMA, 1999;281:2091-7)

Another study on Hormonal Factors in Breast Cancer found that the average length of time a woman takes HRT is 11 years, and that the risk of breast cancer increases by 2.3% for every year of use. Using HRT for five years or more raised the risk of breast cancer by 35%. (Lancet,1997;350:1047-59).

Deciding news from the JAMA

Then in July 2002 the news hit media headlines all over the western world that HRT causes breast cancer, strokes, cardiovascular disease and pulmonary embolism.[75] The study from the Women's Health Initiative that had set out to assess the major health benefits of HRT (oestrogen and progestin) was stopped after five years because, "Overall health risks exceeded benefits... the risk-benefit profile found in this trial is not consistent with the requirements for a viable intervention for primary prevention of chronic disease, and the results indicate that this regimen should not be initiated or continued for primary prevention of CHD (coronary heart disease)."

In other words, although the researchers set out to discover just how good HRT would be in preventing cardiovascular disease, they found that not only were those on the medication experiencing more cardiovascular problems than controls, but also that HRT was causing other major health problems. The study, which used conjugated equine estrogens (as found in Premarin) and medroxyprogesterone (synthetic progestogen as found in Provera) recorded higher than expected rates of pulmonary embolism, cardiovascular disease, strokes and invasive breast cancer. The trial was brought to a halt because it was not considered ethical to continue with such damaging results to women's health.

Background information on HRT

In "Natural Woman, Natural Menopause", Marcus Laux ND and Christine Conrad give an excellent account of the multi-billion dollar HRT industry and how menopause has been 'created' as a hormone deficiency disease by drug companies wanting to offload their products. They go into great detail about the production of one of the most widely prescribed oestrogen replacements, Premarin, as described below.[76]

Premarin, the world's best selling oestrogen replacement product, is made from mare's (female horse) urine. The mares are kept all their lives in stalls too small to turn around in or to lie down. They are kept in perpetual pregnancy and have a catheter to their bladder which is painful for them. When the foals are born, most are disposed of as a useless by-product of the process. To date, it is estimated that half a million horses have stood in concrete stalls and one million foals have been slaughtered to keep up the production of Premarin. The problem with Premarin, besides ethical considerations, is that while it contains some human identical oestrogens like oestrone and oestradiol, it also contains equilin and equilenin (horse oestrogens) and synthetic additives. These substances are not natural to the human female body and cause biochemical confusion that can lead to harmful side effects.

Menopause without HRT

Millions of women before us have been through the menopause without HRT, and millions still do in some parts of the world. They haven't all developed heart disease or osteoporosis. In many parts of the world, particularly Asia, when women follow their traditional diet, they have no incidence of hot flushes and other menopausal symptoms. Nor do they develop heart disease and osteoporosis, despite eating a low calcium diet.

Preventing cardiovascular disease and osteoporosis

It's true that oestrogen helps to keep the artery walls elastic and free from plaque. But having a thyroid that functions adequately is just as important as having high levels of oestrogen, if not more so. Also important are:

- Having sufficient vitamin C for arterial elasticity (1000 mg for daily maintenance)
- Eating enough foods that contain omega-3 fatty acids to keep cholesterol flowing freely
- Taking sufficient exercise, rest and relaxation
- Avoiding free radical damage caused by exposure to environmental pollution, too much alcohol, caffeine, sugar and smoking

In chapter 10 you will see that there are many more factors to consider than just the presence of oestrogen for the prevention of osteoporosis.

Natural HRT following surgical menopause

There are some cases where hormone replacement may be essential, for example after a radical hysterectomy (includes removal of ovaries) when a woman can be plunged into an almost immediate menopause (surgical menopause). In that case, there are balanced hormone replacements based on a the three different kinds of oestrogen: oestradiol, oestrone and oestriol. One such product, Tri-est, is made up of one part oestradiol, one part oestrone and eight parts oestriol and was developed by Dr. Jonathan Wright who has been using oestriol since the 1980s. In his paper *"Don't let your doctor give you horse urine!"*[77], Dr. Wright compares Premarin, containing mare's oestrogens, with human oestrogens, pointing out that *"Premarin produces 'estrogenic effects' which are much more potent and longer lasting than those produced by natural human estrogens."*

But if oestriol is so good and doesn't cause the problems associated with equine oestrogens, why isn't it routinely available and prescribed? The answer, Dr. Wright says, is because it is not patentable, therefore drug companies will not reap the same sort of profits as can be made from other types of HRT.

If you have been prescribed HRT because of surgical menopause, you might want to ask your medical practitioner if you can experiment with Tri-Est and natural progesterone cream or gel. Even if you are taking HRT for 'normal' menopausal symptoms, you might want to see if Tri-Est balanced with natural progesterone would do the job just as well, without the risk of side effects normally associated with conventionally prescribed HRT.

And just in case you are still not convinced …

Risks associated with taking HRT

- Endometrial (lining of the uterus) cancer
- Breast cancer
- Gall stones (rare) but 2 to 3 times greater risk on HRT
- Heart attack – the risk applies to combined oestrogen and progestogen HRT
- Benign liver tumours (rare) that can rupture and bleed into the abdomen
- Elevated blood pressure
- Thrombosis (rare), but especially following surgery
- Thrombophlebitis (inflammation of the wall of a vein)

- Stroke (rare)
- Increase in blood sugar and insulin levels – women with diabetes should be cautious about taking HRT
- Reduced carbohydrate tolerance
- Fluid retention – women who suffer from epilepsy, heart disease, asthma or kidney disease are more at risk on HRT
- Depression – caution for women with a history of depression, or who suffered from depression on the Pill
- Increase in size of fibroids – some types of fibroids increase rapidly on HRT
- Jaundice – applies to women who suffered from jaundice during pregnancy.
- Increased calcium in the blood – women with kidney disease may have problems excreting excess calcium in the blood caused by HRT
- Increase in blood fats and LDLs ('bad' cholesterol) and suppression of HDLs ('good' cholesterol)
- Vitamin B6 and folic acid deficiency. B6 is important in combating menopausal symptoms. Folic acid is required for normal cell division and therefore for the prevention of cancer. Folic acid is helpful in reversing abnormal pre-cancerous cells of the cervix.
- Vaginal spotting and break-through bleeding
- Vision disturbance (rare) caused by progestogens
- Virilisation – increase in facial hair and deepening voice
- Risk for smokers – women taking HRT should not smoke due to the increased harmful effects on heart and blood vessels
- Breast tenderness and swelling
- Headaches and migraine
- Abdominal cramps
- Hair loss, skin rashes, nausea, backache, anxiety
- Weight gain – sudden increase often with a noticeable increase in breast size
- Cystitis-like symptoms

Nutrition first

With a list of negative potential side effects and risk from taking HRT, women should ask themselves if it is really worth taking the risk when there are perfectly good natural alternatives. True, modifying your diet and lifestyle may take more effort, but the only side effect will be an increase in health and the 'feel good' factor.

CHAPTER 10
LOSS OF BONE DENSITY AND OSTEOPOROSIS

Your living skeleton

You can have a lot of influence over bone health through your dietary and lifestyle choices. Bones are living and changing organisms in the body. The skeleton you have now is not the same skeleton you had ten years ago, nor the same one you will have in ten years' time. Bones are made up of a collagen (form of protein) matrix which provides the framework for calcium and other minerals in crystal form. Osteoclasts and osteoblasts are the cells at bone ends that control the regeneration of bone with osteoclasts breaking down old bone to make way for osteoblasts to form new bone. Bone strength is affected by a complex interaction between several hormones and the presence (or absence) of a wide range of vitamins and minerals.[78]

We all know that bones need calcium. But that's only a small part of the story. Besides calcium, bones require vitamins A, B6, C, D, E, K, folic acid, magnesium, manganese, boron, strontium, silicon, zinc and copper in trace amounts for their health and strength. Calcium and magnesium are macro minerals, meaning that they are needed in larger quantities. As well as bone strength, calcium and magnesium fulfil many other functions in the body, including a role in the immune system, the transfer of electrical messages via the nervous system, and muscle contraction and relaxation. Bones provide a good storage depot for these minerals and they can be called upon to top up levels of calcium and magnesium when blood levels fall. The passage of calcium and magnesium in and out of the bones is controlled by two hormones, parathyroid hormone and calcitonin.

Parathyroid hormone causes calcium to be taken from the bones in response to low levels of circulating calcium in the blood. Its other jobs are to stimulate the action of osteoclasts (the cells that break down old bone) to activate vitamin D, which in turn ensures calcium is absorbed from food through the intestine wall, and to reduce the amount of calcium lost via the kidneys in urine.

Oestrogen plays a role in the regulation of parathyroid hormone. Too little oestrogen results in too much parathyroid hormone (hyperparathyroidism) with a corresponding increase in bone turnover. A lack of oestrogen also stops vitamin D activity which results in less formation of bone matrix.

Secreted from cells in the thyroid, calcitonin balances the action of parathyroid hormone. When there is adequate calcium in the blood, calcitonin lays down calcium in the bones. Besides stopping the release of calcium from the bones, it also stimulates the action of osteoblasts, the bone building cells.

Stress and menopause

Busy women with too much to do and under stress produce more of the stress hormone, cortisol, which also plays a part in bone density. Cortisol's job is to increase the sensitivity of bone cells to parathyroid hormone, vitamin D and growth factors.[79] At low doses, i.e. when there is no particular stress, cortisol stimulates osteoblasts to form new bone, whereas high cortisol levels increase the breakdown of bone. In effect, stress causes more rapid bone breakdown.

Stress combined with menopause is a particularly potent mixture as far as bones are concerned. Normally oestrogen helps keep levels of cortisol low, but as oestrogen levels decline during and after menopause, cortisol levels can rise unchecked, leading to more loss of bone density. But not all postmenopausal women suffer from osteoporosis. This is partly because nature has provided a safety mechanism for menopausal bones. In men, osteoblasts are stimulated by androgens (male hormones), and in particular testosterone. In postmenopausal women with healthy adrenal glands, as oestrogen levels drop, increased levels of androgens are produced in the adrenals, thus providing a safeguard against excessive bone loss. The key to bone health is, therefore, to maintain healthy adrenal glands through good nutrition and good stress management.

Osteoporosis

Osteoporosis, as defined by the World Health Organisation (WHO), is when bone density decreases and the bones become brittle, fragile and easily broken. According to the National Osteoporosis Society in the UK, 1 in 3 women will develop osteoporosis severe enough to cause a fracture. Internationally more than 1.5 million fractures occur every year (primarily of the hips, vertebrae or wrists) as a result of osteoporosis. While the majority of people who suffer from osteoporosis are postmenopausal women, bone mass begins to decline at 35 years of age, and then accelerates rapidly for eight to ten years around the time of menopause. Thereafter, bone loss continues at a slower rate.[80]

Osteoporosis is no longer confined to women. Men are also being affected by loss of bone density, with estimates being as high as 1 in 12 men suffering from fractures due to osteoporosis. These statistics present a rather gloomy picture and medical science is searching for answers to reverse the trend.

Symptoms and risk factors

Osteoporosis is a silent disease because there are no obvious symptoms. The first sign people know there is something wrong is when they break a bone, often in the wrist or spine, following a minor bump or fall. Osteoporosis also causes the small vertebrae in the spine to crush or wedge, often causing chronic pain and curvature of the spine which results in a loss of height and a hump in the back (dowager's hump).

The people most at risk from osteoporosis are postmenopausal caucasian and oriental women over the age of 50. U.S. demographics show that people of African descent have higher bone mass and lower rates of fractures, while in Europe the highest rates of vertebral deformities are in Scandinavian countries.[81]

Other risk factors for both men and women are:

• Early menopause or early hysterectomy (especially if both ovaries are removed), before age 45
• Family history of osteoporosis or maternal history of hip fracture
• History of over active thyroid
• Hypercalciuria (abnormally high amounts of calcium in the urine)
• Medications: long term use of steroids, e.g. for asthma, dilantin, thyroid hormone, heparin, gonadotrophin releasing hormone agonists, anticonvulsants and benzodiazepines
• Liver disease
• Long term immobility
• Malabsorption due to low stomach acid, inflammatory bowel disease and gastric surgery
• Moderate to high alcohol and caffeine intake and smoking
• Low body weight and anorexia leading to a reduction in oestrogen levels

Testing for bone density

The safest and most accurate ways to measure bone density are with Photon Absorptionmetry and Dual Energy X-ray Absorptionmetry (DEXA), the latter being 96%-98% accurate and using very low dose x-rays. Dr. Lee recommends that women at risk for osteoporosis have a bone mineral density measurement as they are going into menopause. That way they have a base line with which to compare later bone density tests.[82] He also recommends measuring height every six months to monitor loss of height – a sure sign that bone is being lost on the spine.

Drugs to treat osteoporosis

There are a number of different drugs being used for the treatment of low bone mineral density. Bisphosphonates are non-hormonal drugs that work by inhibiting osteoclastic activity, thereby halting the breakdown of old bone. Bisphosphonates, such as Didronel and Fosamax, have to be used with caution as constant daily use can cause abnormalities in bone mineralisation.[83] They are taken on a cyclical basis for a limited number of years. The side effects from taking Fosamax, as listed in the British National Formulary, are quite impressive and include severe oesophageal (food pipe) reactions such as inflammation, ulcers, stricture and erosions. The rest of the digestive tract can also be affected with symptoms such as abdominal pain and distension, diarrhoea or constipation, flatulence, musculoskeletal pain, and more rarely vomiting, peptic ulcers and photosensitivity. According to Dr. Lee, the drawback with bisphosphonates is that the old bone they save is *"eventually unsound, and after three or four years they have no benefit."* They therefore do not offer a long term solution to osteoporosis.

Other drugs used to treat osteoporosis are the hormones calcitrol (an active form of vitamin D) and calcitonin (to slow down osteoclast activity), usually by muscle injection or nasal spray. Testosterone for male osteoporosis, anabolic steroids for the frail and elderly to build bone and muscle mass, and SERMs (Selective Estrogen Receptor Modulators), a new generation of synthetic hormone replacement, are also used to treat osteoporosis. While apparently helpful for the time they are taken, all of the above carry lists of side effects and have to be used with caution. In any case, apart from calcitrol (vitamin D), none of them addresses the underlying nutritional deficiencies associated with the development of osteoporosis.

HRT and calcium

Besides the above, other mainstream treatment for osteoporosis includes HRT (usually a combination of oestrogen and progestogen) and high doses of calcium. Because oestrogen is important in regulating the action of parathyroid hormone, (thereby slowing down the rate of bone breakdown and calcium release from the bones), it is assumed that the main reason menopausal women get osteoporosis is because of a drop in oestrogen levels. The simple solution is therefore to provide oestrogen. But there are drawbacks. It is true that HRT can slow down the rate of destruction of old bone, but it cannot completely halt it. And once HRT is discontinued, the rate of bone destruction speeds up dramatically in a 'catch up' way. According to a large study published in the New England Journal of Medicine in 1995 that followed over 9,500 women, oestrogen therapy was shown to be protective in those women without a history of osteoporosis or fracture, but after five to six years, bone loss continues at the same rate, with or without oestrogen.[84]

Now, with HRT receiving such bad press, many women are going to be reluctant to trade short term increased bone density for invasive breast cancer, pulmonary embolism, strokes and cardiovascular disease. In any case, tackling osteoporosis with oestrogen-progestogen replacement completely ignores all the complexities of bone destruction and regeneration, and all the factors that influence this ongoing process from cradle to grave. It does nothing to tackle the real causes of loss of bone density which include:

• Processed and 'fast' food
• Moderate to high consumption of salt, sugar, caffeine and alcohol
• Smoking
• Nutritional deficiencies
• Low stomach acid
• Sedentary lifestyle and lack of exercise
• High stress levels

How much calcium?

Giving calcium in the form of supplements to women with low bone density or osteoporosis seems logical enough. After all the body contains more calcium than any other mineral with about 99 per cent being concentrated in bones and teeth. Around 10 grams is needed in the rest of the body to regulate heart beat, nerve transmissions, muscle contraction, and blood coagulation. Calcium also plays a part in controlling blood acid/alkaline balance, cell division, muscle growth and iron utilisation. The calcium found in bones is in the form of calcium phosphate.

But there is more to having the right amount of calcium in the bones than just taking calcium supplements. In his book, "*Trace elements, hair analysis and nutrition*", Richard Passwater, PhD points out that calcium balance is a complex process that depends on many different factors, including absorption from food. Calcium absorption starts in the stomach where stomach acid splits the calcium from its protein carrier.[85] Once released from food, calcium travels to the small intestine where it is absorbed through the intestinal wall into the blood.

However, not all the calcium you eat is absorbed. Calcium absorption efficiency varies according to the amount available and what is required by the body. Someone who is deficient in calcium will be much more efficient at absorbing it through their intestine than someone who eats plenty. High calcium consumers tend to absorb less and excrete more in faeces. This has made it difficult to set exact amounts of calcium required for health. The current RDA (recommended daily allowance) in the U.S. is 1200 mg. In the EC (European Community) it is 800 mg, while according to Dr. Passwater, the World Health Organisation noted in 1962 that man has the ability to adapt to wide ranges of calcium intake and that intakes vary widely from country to country. Because a range of 300 to 1000 mg seems to work in different cultures, a *"practical allowance"* of 400 to 500 mg per day is suggested.

People who are under stress or in an anxiety state use up calcium much faster than when they are not stressed as their calcium can become tied up as calcium lactate. Pregnant and lactating women also have a higher need for calcium, with recommended amounts of around 1200 to 1400 mg.

Not all calcium supplements are equal

Calcium is the most abundant mineral found in the bones and it is the loss of calcium that results in osteoporosis. This has led to women being prescribed very high doses of calcium (1000 – 1200 mg) to slow down this depletion from the bones. The form of calcium prescribed is usually calcium carbonate which is not very well utilised or absorbed in the body in large quantities. Excess calcium carbonate not absorbed into the bone is excreted via the kidneys. When the quantity exceeds the body's ability to excrete calcium, it gets deposited in soft tissue and joints, leading to arthritic changes and joint pain. It can also stay in the kidneys where it can cause kidney stones.[86]

Joan's story

Joan wanted advice about the menopause. She had been prescribed HRT and calcium by her doctor because a bone density scan had revealed a slight decrease in bone density in her spine. After taking the calcium supplements for about six months, Joan developed joint pain in her wrists and ankles - although she hadn't associated the calcium supplement with her pain. When she stopped the high levels of calcium carbonate and instead took a more balanced supplement with magnesium, the joint aches and pains eventually stopped.

Better forms of calcium are calcium citrate and calcium citrate malate. Studies have shown that calcium citrate is better absorbed than calcium carbonate and provides greater bone protective effects than calcium carbonate. Calcium citrate has also been shown to be helpful in preventing the formation of kidney stones, a potential danger of taking calcium carbonate supplements. The citrate binds with calcium in the urine, reducing the amount available to form calcium oxalate crystals. It also reduces acidity in the urine which inhibits the development of both calcium oxalate and uric acid stones.[87] Because of its bioavailability, more calcium citrate is absorbed from supplements than calcium carbonate, meaning less can be used to greater effect.

Is osteoporosis really a calcium deficiency disease?

While women are being told they need more calcium and should take supplements or drink plenty of milk, it is clear that creating healthy bones isn't as straightforward as that. While some studies have been done to show that postmenopausal women need more calcium due to higher urinary excretion of calcium and poorer ability to absorb calcium, others show that most people with osteoporosis *do not* have a calcium deficiency. Dr. John McLaren Howard of BioLab Medical Unit in the U.K. looked at the nutritional profiles of a number of patients with osteoporosis and compared them with controls, menstruating women, postmenopausal women with no osteoporosis and postmenopausal women on HRT. Results showed that none of the women studied, whether they had osteoporosis or were taking HRT, had low calcium levels.[88] Another study showed that only 25% of women with osteoporosis had low calcium levels, the other 75% gaining no benefit from taking calcium supplements,[89] and yet another showed that increased calcium intake does not prevent early postmenopausal bone loss.[90]

What BioLab did discover was that women with osteoporosis lacked many other nutrients important for bone formation, as well as the bone enzyme, alkaline phosphatase. This enzyme, activated by magnesium, helps to form calcium crystals in the bone. It therefore serves as a good indicator of whether new bone is being laid down or not. The study showed that the lowest levels of alkaline phosphatase were in the women with osteoporosis on HRT.

Magnesium is important too

These studies highlight the importance of magnesium in preventing osteoporosis. Because magnesium is necessary to activate alkaline phosphatase, another researcher, Dr. Guy Abrahams, believes that magnesium rather than calcium deficiency is responsible for osteoporosis. Dr. Abraham conducted a trial of magnesium therapy in 26 postmenopausal women, all taking either oestrogen alone or oestrogen plus a progestogen. They were given dietary advice that included avoiding processed foods, emphasizing vegetable over animal protein, limiting salt, sugar, alcohol, coffee, tea, chocolate and tobacco intake. Each participant also received a daily supplement containing 600 mg of magnesium (oxide) and 500 mg of calcium (citrate), an unconventionally high magnesium to calcium ratio. The supplement also contained vitamin C, B-vitamins, vitamin D, zinc, copper, manganese, boron, and other nutrients.[91] Bone density studies before and eight to nine months after the start of the study showed an average increase in bone density of 11% in those taking the magnesium and other supplements, compared to only 0.7% in those who received hormone replacement alone, a significant increase in a relatively short space of time.

The milk myth

And what about milk for calcium? So many women assure me that they are drinking milk and eating dairy produce to prevent osteoporosis. They are under-standably shocked when they learn that women who drink the most milk suffer the most bone breakages, and the countries that consume the most diary products have the highest rates of osteoporosis!

So what is going on here?

Milk and dairy produce consumption in the West is one of the greatest marketing success stories of our time so that most women believe that they must have milk products to ensure adequate calcium intake to prevent osteoporosis. This is completely untrue. Fully grown wild animals do not eat dairy produce or drink milk (and neither do they get osteoporosis!). Milk is a food for baby animals, not for fully grown human beings. No other species suckles milk from another species, and no other species continues to drink milk past the age of weaning, apart from human beings.

According to Dr. John McDougall, member of PCRM (The Physicians Committee for Responsible Medicine),[92] a 1985 study funded by the U.S. National Dairy Council involved giving a group of postmenopausal women three 8 oz (236 ml) glasses of skimmed milk per day for one year and comparing their bones to those of a control group of women not given any milk. The dairy group were consuming 1,400 mg of calcium per day and lost bone at twice the rate of the control group. Because the results *"did not reach statistical significance"* the researchers concluded that 24 oz (709 ml) or three glasses of milk per day had no effect on bones, thereby evading the real truth of the experiment. Since then no other clinical trials have been carried out on the benefits of milk consumption, presumably because it is accepted that milk does not stop bones breaking.

Dr. Walter Willett, a veteran nutrition researcher at the Harvard School of Public Health, says that calcium consumption has become like *"a religious crusade, overshadowing true preventive measures against osteoporosis."* He took part in the famous Harvard Nurses Health study that followed over 70,000 women for a 12-year period and found that milk did not protect against bone fractures. In fact, those women who drank three glasses of milk per day had more fractures than those who rarely drank milk.[93] An Australian study showed the same results.[94]

Finally, the American Journal of Clinical Nutrition concluded, *"the body of scientific evidence appears inadequate to support a recommendation for daily intake of dairy foods to promote bone health in the general U.S. public."*[95]

Several studies have been done linking milk products with an increased risk of ovarian cancer in lactose (milk sugar) intolerant women. Galactose, one of the sugars in lactose, is toxic to the ovaries and can interfere with fertility. Some researchers believe that it may even cause birth defects and cataracts.[96,97,98]

What's wrong with milk?

The problems with milk are many. Dairy products, such as milk and cheese, contain high amounts of calcium, but low amounts of magnesium, which is important for the activation of alkaline phosphatase. Thus you get a very high ratio of calcium to magnesium, which can lead to increased urinary loss of magnesium.

Most dairy products, including milk, but especially cheese, also contain significant amounts of sodium. Sodium causes urinary calcium loss, meaning literally peeing away calcium, especially if you consume significant amounts of other highly salted processed foods like breads, snack foods, processed meats, soya products, and junk food.

Milk fat acts as a storage depot for toxins, such as pesticides and organochlorines, dioxins, antibiotics and hormones that are either naturally present in the animal's milk, or have been added as a growth enhancer. Antibiotics are routinely given to cattle to promote growth and protect them from diseases prophylactically (to prevent rather than cure disease). The pesticide Lindane, still being used in the UK but banned in Israel, has been linked with an increased risk of breast cancer in agricultural areas where it is sprayed. It is particularly found in dairy products, such as milk, butter and cheese.[99]

Dairy products are highly allergic for a lot of people, causing digestive problems, ear, throat and nose infections and sinusitis. Most women have a slight, clear vaginal discharge which normally causes no problem. Women who suffer from a mucousy or heavy white discharge requiring protection with light pads, tell me that it usually clears up when they stop using dairy products, indicating a sensitivity to dairy produce. If you suspect you may have a dairy produce allergy, have a go at the allergy pulse test described in chapter 7.

Fermented and organic

That said, not all women react badly to dairy products. If you have no sensitivity and you enjoy the taste, fermented milk products such as yoghurt and cottage cheese are better bets for calcium. The calcium has already been pre-digested by fermenting bacteria and is therefore more readily absorbed through the intestinal wall.[100] It is important to choose organically produced yoghurt and cottage cheese to reduce the risk of hormone, antibiotic and pesticide contamination. Also choose yoghurts that contain live bacteria and no sugar. Avoid drinking milk or adding it to cereals. You can find alternatives to milk in chapter 11.

Alternative food sources of calcium

All the nutrients needed for bone health are found in whole, unprocessed foods, grown on composted fertile soils, without the aid of pesticides, herbicides and artificial fertilizers. Food processing, particularly the refining of grains, removes between 70% and 90% of vitamins, minerals, essential fatty acids and fibre – all of which are important for hormone and bone health. As many people rely heavily on refined wheat based foods as their staple diet (pasta, bread, breakfast cereals, sandwiches, pizzas, cakes, biscuits), the deficit in valuable nutrients can soon mount up.

Organic crops contain significantly more vitamin C, iron, magnesium, and phosphorus and significantly less nitrates than conventional crops. Organic fruit and vegetables also have a higher content of nutritionally significant minerals and lower amounts of some heavy metals compared to conventionally grown produce. There appears to be genuine differences in the nutrient content of organic and conventional crops.[101,102] It's certainly worth buying organic where you can and if you are a keen gardener with room to spare, start growing at least some of your own!

Table 2 shows the calcium content of fruit, vegetables, oily fish, seeds and nuts and the spreads made with them, dried fruit, pulses (dried beans, peas and lentils) and seaweed in comparison with milk products. Seaweed is exceptionally high in calcium as well as all other minerals and is an excellent source of phytohormones.

Fruit and vegetables	Mg of calcium per cupful (cooked)
Apricots (8 dried apricots)	46
Broccoli	94-177
Brussels sprouts	56
Green cabbage	50
Carrot	48
Cauliflower	34
Celery (raw) 1 stalk	14
Chinese cabbage(bok choy cooked)	148-357
Dandelion greens	104
French beans	111
Figs (4 dried figs)	168
Kale	94-179
Lettuce (iceberg)	15
Onions	104
Peas (frozen)	38
Pepper (green, raw)	6
Potatoes baked with skin 1 large	40
Pumpkin	74
Spinach	244
Turnip greens	194-249
Watercress (raw)	40

Seaweed	Mg of calcium per cupful (cooked)
Agar agar (dry flakes)	400
Dulse	570
Kelp	610
Wakame	520

Pulses and legumes	Mg of calcium per cupful (cooked)
Baked beans (200 g)	90
Chick peas	150
Kidney beans (canned)	69
Navy beans	123
Pinto beans	130
Soya beans	130
Split peas	52

Soya products	Mg of calcium in 112 gms
Soya cheese (40g slice)	180
Tempeh	170
Tofu precipitated with calcium salts	300
Tofu soya bean curd	100

Nuts and seeds	Mg of calcium per cup
Almonds	300
Almond butter (1 tablespoon)	86
Brazil nuts	260
Hazelnuts	282
Pine nuts	28
Sesame seeds	148
Sunflower seeds	132
Tahini (sesame paste - 1 tablespoon)	64
Walnuts	108

Fish	Mg of calcium per 125 gm serving
Bass, baked	7
Herring, baked	95
Lobster, steamed	78
Mackerel, baked	20
Oysters (4 large raw oysters)	196
Perch, baked	45
Prawns	130
Salmon, canned	271
Sardines, canned in oil	92
Swordfish, baked	101
Tuna, canned in oil	109

Dairy products (for comparison)	Mg of calcium per cup
Cheese (per 25 gm serving)	200
Cottage cheese (45 g)	33
Low fat cheese	150
Milk	300
Non-fat yoghurt	295
Skimmed milk	285

Table 2. Calcium content of food in comparison with dairy products

Foods that promote calcium loss

Some foods actively promote the excretion of calcium, particularly the acid forming foods. Blood is normally alkaline, having a pH of around 7.5. All fruit, vegetables, seeds and almonds have an alkalising effect on the blood, even citrus fruits. All the rest, i.e. meat, fish, eggs, cheese, cereals, sugar, bread, pasta, rice, alcohol, coffee, tea, cola drinks, chocolate and tobacco, raise blood acidity. The body uses calcium and magnesium to neutralise too much acid meaning that people who eat too many acid forming foods use up more calcium than is available circulating in the blood. Detecting a drop in blood levels of calcium, the parathyroid stimulates the release of calcium from the bones to neutralise the acidity. The net result is an overall drop in calcium in the bones.

Not all the acid-forming foods should be avoided. Grains, meat, fish, eggs, pulses, bread, nuts and vinegar are all perfectly normal and healthy foods (providing there is no food intolerance). The important thing is to maintain a balance, the ideal balance being around 70% alkalising foods with the remaining 30% taken from the acid forming foods.

Acid-forming foods	Exceptions, i.e. they are alkalising
All grains, e.g. wheat, oats, rye, buckwheat and rice	Millet , quinoa
Foods made with flour, especially white flour	
Breakfast cereals and bread (all kinds)	Unless made with millet or quinoa
All meat, poultry, seafood and fish, including bacon	
Milk products, including cheese	Milk and butter are regarded as neutral
Eggs	
Pulses (beans, peas, lentils, soya beans and tofu) and peanuts	
Nuts	Almonds
Vinegar	
Sugar, alcohol, coffee and smoking	

Alkaline-forming Foods	Exceptions
Fruit (including citrus fruits and dried fruit) Vegetables (including seaweed and potatoes) Seeds, e.g. pumpkin, sesame, sunflower and linseed Millet, quinoa and almonds Mineral water Ginseng, ginger, mustard, pepper, curry, most spices	

Table. 3 Acid and alkaline promoting foods
Adapted from "The Optimum Nutrition Bible" by Patrck Holford

Foods to avoid

It is important to note that some foods should be kept strictly for occasional use only, or avoided completely by women who have existing osteoporosis.

- Foods made with white, refined flour
- Sugar and anything made with it
- Caffeine
- Alcohol
- Chocolate
- Salt
- Fizzy / cola drinks
- Smoking

Refined foods, sugar, caffeine, alcohol and chocolate are highly acid forming and therefore cause loss of calcium and magnesium.

Salt

While it hasn't been conclusively proved that salt consumption increases bone loss, some studies show that increased dietary salt causes an increase in urine excretion of calcium.[103] It may therefore be wise to cut down on salt in food, and especially avoid highly salted snacks such as crisps (potato chips), salted nuts and snack biscuits. Prepared meals and restaurant food also contain high amounts of salt and should not be relied on for daily nutrition.

Fizzy drinks

Fizzy (carbonated) drinks contain phosphoric acid to "buffer" their acidity. Some reports show that young cola drinkers have an increased incidence of bone fractures.[104] Children drinking at least six glasses of fizzy drinks containing phosphoric acid had more than five times the risk of developing low blood levels of calcium compared to other children.[105] Avoiding fizzy drinks containing phosphoric acid also seems to reduce the formation of kidney stones, probably because of the link to abnormal calcium metabolism.[106]

This does not apply to naturally sparkling mineral water which makes a refreshing alternative to sweetened fizzy drinks, alcohol, tea or coffee. Don't be tempted by mineral waters that have added calcium (usually calcium carbonate) or those that have been flavoured (they are usually sweetened and coloured). You can flavour your own with a dash of lemon juice, some squeezed ginger, or half and half fruit juice and mineral water.

Coffee

A large study that followed American women for six years found that those who drank two to three cups, or more, of coffee per day lost more calcium in their urine than those who were not coffee drinkers. The results were particularly significant in women who had a low calcium intake to start with. The authors of the study recommended that women reduce or avoid caffeine from caffeinated coffee, black tea and cola drinks.[107,108,109] Chocolate also contains caffeine, so should be kept to a minimum.

Protein

Plenty of conflicting research has been done on the effect of excessive amounts of protein and, conversely too little protein, in connection with an increased risk for osteoporosis.[110,111] Researchers are confused about the link between increased amounts of phosphorous found especially in animal protein and the ratio between calcium and phosphorous needed to make healthy bones (bones are made up of calcium phosphate, derived from phosphorous).

What seems clear is that, as in all things, balance is the key. Bones need a certain level of protein to build the protein matrix that provides the framework upon which calcium and other minerals adhere. Women are consuming either too little or too much protein, too many other acid-forming foods including junk food and snacks, and insufficient alkalising fruit, vegetables, seeds and almonds. The Seven Day Meal Planner (chapter 17) gives you a good idea of balanced meals with optimum amounts of protein and based around whole, unrefined foods, with no salty or fatty snacks, caffeine, alcohol, fizzy drinks, sugar or milk, and only small amounts of unrefined sea salt for extra minerals and iodine.

Beware fluoride!

If you thought fluoride was a harmless substance added to water supplies and toothpaste to prevent tooth decay, think again! Fluoride is hazardous waste from the nuclear arms, aluminium, glass production and phosphate fertiliser industries. It is also a rat poison.

"Fluoride is more poisonous than lead, and just less poisonous than arsenic" (Clinical Toxicology of Commercial Products 1984)

"A seven ounce tube of toothpaste, theoretically at least, contains enough fluoride to kill a small child." Procter & Gamble.

Dr. Dean Burk of the U.S. National Cancer Institute summed up the nature of fluoride in his statement, *"Fluoride causes more human cancer death, and causes it faster than any other chemical."*[112]

As far as bones are concerned, fluoride interferes with the mineralisation of bones leading to abnormal bone density and bone that lacks tensile strength. It causes osteoporosis by creating a calcium deficiency state as well as the build up of calcium stones and crystals in the joints and organs. Fluoride causes a wide variety of health problems from cancer to osteoporosis and premature ageing due to its ability to interfere with enzyme systems, proteins and quite probably DNA itself.[113]

Avoid fluoridated dental products and filter all your tap water for making hot drinks, cooking rice, potatoes, pasta and vegetables. Use a water filter that guarantees to remove fluoride. This is especially important if you live in an area where the public water supply is routinely fluoridated.

Oxalic and phytic acid

Oxalic and phytic acids are naturally occurring substances found in some foods. Oxalic acid is present in rhubarb, spinach, and cocoa (and therefore chocolate). Phytic acid is found in raw, whole grains, for example those used to make mueslis. Both have the ability to bind up minerals, including calcium, in the intestine and hinder their absorption. This in itself is not normally a problem in people with adequate calcium status, but if you are at risk of (or already have) osteoporosis, be sure to soak your muesli overnight or eat cooked grains to neutralise phytic acid. Keep cocoa products to a minimum and don't eat spinach or rhubarb every day!

Chocolate for magnesium?

Women tell me that it's OK to eat chocolate because it contains magnesium, which is true, chocolate does contain magnesium. But apart from the high sugar, fat and caffeine content, chocolate also contains oxalic acid which makes the magnesium much less absorbable. In any case, chocolate is a stimulant which means that it stresses the adrenal glands and causes the loss of magnesium (chapter 13). So don't kid yourself you are boosting magnesium levels by eating chocolate! Much better to get your magnesium from seeds and nuts.

Stomach acid

No amount of calcium, good food or mineral supplements will improve bone density if there is insufficient stomach acid. Acid in the stomach is there to break down protein in food. As all minerals come in nature attached to a protein, in order for them to be released for absorption in the intestine, there has to be sufficient stomach acid to break down their protein carrier and set them free.

The first thing a woman suffering from osteoporosis must do is to check for low stomach acid. There are laboratory tests that can be done, but I have found the simplest, cheapest and most effective way is to take a capsule or tablet of betaine hydrochloride, similar to your own stomach acid. Supplements of betaine hydrochloride are often complexed with pepsin to help break down protein and are available from good health food shops. Take the supplement with a main meal containing protein (not with a light snack or breakfast). Monitor how you feel. If there is no warm sensation within 20 minutes to a couple of hours after taking the supplement, it's a sign that you could do with some extra stomach acid. You then need to continue taking betaine hydrochloride at each main meal that contains protein, along with a good multi vitamin and mineral supplement containing zinc and vitamin B6 to help encourage your stomach to produce the correct amount of acid. When stomach acid levels have normalised, anywhere between one and six months later, you will feel a warm or prickly sensation in the stomach after taking the supplement. That is the sign to stop the supplements.

As levels of stomach acid tend to fall with age, it may be worth while for all women to check that they are producing enough, especially if they suffer from digestive problems and feelings of indigestion (chapter 14).

Sandra's story

Sandra was a lady in her fifties with loss of bone density and bone and joint pain. Her diet was excellent and she used to enjoy a regular game of tennis, although this had become difficult with her joint pain. On the recommendation of a Belgian sports specialist, she took an optimum range of good quality supplements, including calcium, magnesium and vitamin D. Her continuing bone problems, despite an excellent diet and high quality supplements, were a dilemma until I suggested that she had a test for stomach acid, which she had done at a laboratory in England. The results were conclusive – she was producing insufficient stomach acid to absorb the minerals, including calcium, from her food and her supplements. After taking betaine hydrochloride for four to five months, Sandra's symptoms started to improve, she regained mobility and had less joint pain. She was delighted at being able to play a game of pain-free tennis again.

Digestive enzymes

Women who have difficulty digesting fats often do well when they take a supplement of digestive enzymes that contains lipase, a fat digesting enzyme. If after doing the stomach acid test you find that you need more stomach acid, I recommend taking betaine hydrochloride with a course of digestive enzymes to ensure that you are getting the most effective absorption of nutrients from your healthy diet as possible. Avoid digestive enzymes that contain animal products such as pancreatin and ox bile, which can cause a reaction in some people.

Your bones need more than calcium

It seems clear that although HRT and calcium can slow down the rate of osteoporosis in some cases, they cannot stop it, and they certainly cannot reverse it. If the studies done so far are accurate, then taking calcium supplements may lead to joint problems and kidney stones. In any case, this approach to bone density loss ignores all the other important factors involved in the creation and maintenance of healthy bone, even in postmenopausal women. In the Journal of Nutritional Medicine 1990, Drs Alan Gaby and Jonathan Wright wrote a comprehensive review article of the nutrients related to osteoporosis. They highlight magnesium, vitamins A, B6, C, D and K, zinc, phosphorus and boron as being essential for bone health.[114] The following is taken from their review article.

Vitamin D and magnesium - Don't be afraid of the sun

The most important of these, mainly because most women don't get enough, are magnesium and vitamin D – both of which help to increase calcium uptake and absorption. The most important source of vitamin D is through the action of sunlight on skin and is therefore particularly deficient in sunless northern climates. It can also become a problem for women who spend most of their time working inside. Taking a supplement in the form of fish liver oil provides adequate vitamins A and D during the long, grey winter months that characterise Northern European winters.

When the sun does shine, spend as much time as you can outside taking regular sun baths, building up a gentle tan slowly and without burning the skin. According to Richard Hobday in his book, "*The Healing Sun*", the best time of day for safe tanning is early morning during spring and early summer. He also notes that tanned skin makes more vitamin D in the form of vitamin D3, needed to absorb calcium in the intestines.[115]

Magnesium is needed to activate alkaline phosphatase, an enzyme involved in forming new calcium crystals. It is also needed to convert vitamin D to its active form, 1,25-dihyroxyvitamin D3. Magnesium deficiency has become so common among women due to higher stress levels and food refining that many doctors in Belgium (although alas not yet in the UK) now recognise magnesium deficiency and prescribe it as they would any other medication.

Vitamin K

Vitamin K is usually known for it role in blood clotting. However, it is also required for the synthesis of osteocalcin, a protein found uniquely in large amounts in bone. Osteocalcin is the protein matrix upon which calcium crystallizes. Lack of vitamin K increases excretion of calcium through the kidneys. As this vitamin is normally found in vegetables, people eating fewer than five servings of vegetables per day may not be getting enough vitamin K. Antibiotics also kill off the bacteria in the intestines that normally produce vitamin K. Eating plenty of vegetables and taking a probiotic to rebalance intestinal flora will go a long way towards ensuring adequate vitamin K.

Vitamin B6 and Folic Acid

Both vitamin B6 and folic acid are required for the detoxification of a toxic compound called homocysteine which is produced as a result of the breakdown of the amino acid, methionine, in the body. Too much homocysteine damages

102

artery walls, and bone endings. Vitamin B6 is also a cofactor in the production of collagen which increases the strength of connective tissue in the protein matrix of the bone. Smoking, alcohol, the Pill and HRT reduce B6 and folic acid levels.

Manganese, zinc, strontium, silicon and copper

Manganese is required for bone mineralisation and for the synthesis of connective tissue in cartilage and bone. Manganese deficiency leads to smaller, less dense bones with less resistance to fractures.

Zinc is essential for normal bone formation and for enhancing the biochemical action of vitamin D3.

Strontium is normally assoicated with radioactive strontium, a component of nuclear fallout, that can accumulate in bone tissue. Non-radioactive strontium occurs naturally in food and water, and appears to reduce the incidence of dental caries and bone resorption.

Silicon is found in high concentrations at calcification sites in growing bone. It appears to strengthen the connective tissue matrix by cross-linking collagen strands. Horsetail is a useful herb as it is a rich source of silicon.

Copper is needed for normal bone synthesis as it strengthens connective tissue in the protein matrix.

Boron – natural HRT

Boron is a mineral that deserves a mention here. It has been discovered that between just 1 and 3 mg of boron per day slows down the excretion of calcium in urine and increases naturally occurring oestrogens in the blood, particularly a form of oestradiol. There seems to be no toxicity at these levels of boron. In countries where the diet contains as much as 41 mg of boron per day, no problems have been reported.[116]

Unlike conventional HRT, boron is believed to be able to reduce the risk of cancer due to its ability to increase oestriol levels, a form of oestrogen known to prevent certain types of cancer. All good quality supplements should now contain boron, especially if they are aimed at women.

Regular exercise

Exercise is not an optional extra in a bone maintenance lifestyle. It is essential to bone health. Lack of regular exercise is a major contributory factor in osteoporosis. Recommendation from the National Osteoporosis Society is to exercise at least three times a week for a minimum of 20 minutes. Choose load bearing exercise such as running, skipping, racket sports, dancing, and weight training. Even jumping on the spot 50 times each day can increase bone density in pre-menopausal women.[117]

Exercise keeps calcium in the bones and not deposited in joints and soft tissue. If you can't bear the thought of getting hot and sweaty in a gym, buy yourself a pair of comfortable walking shoes or boots, and start walking! The majority of people can walk. It's cheap, it gets you out of doors and is good all round toning exercise.

Natural progesterone

Dr. John Lee, an American country doctor, is best known for his work using natural progesterone. In her book, *"Passage to Power"*, Leslie Kenton tells us how Dr. Lee treated many of his patients suffering from postmenopausal osteoporosis using natural progesterone cream as part of a programme that involved a healthy diet, vitamin and mineral supplements and regular light exercise. Dr. Lee's results, when published after ten years, showed that not only had his treatment with natural progesterone halted bone loss in his patients, but they had increased bone density by an average of 15%. Those with the worst loss of bone at the start of treatment showed a much greater than average improvement of between 30% and 40% over three years. The incidence of bone fracture among his patients was way below the expected level for post menopausal osteoporosis, and those that did incur fractures through accidents, such as falling down stairs, had healed much more quickly than expected.[118,119]

Essential fatty acids

In one study, the essential fatty acids found in fish oil, notably EPA (eicosapentaenoic acid) and DHA (docosahexaenoic acid), and GLA (gamma linolenic acid) found in evening primrose oil have shown to help improve calcium metabolism. After taking fish oil and evening primrose oil with a 600 mg calcium supplement, women with osteoporosis had a significant 3.1% increase in spinal bone mineral density than control groups.[120,121]

With the advent of hydrogenation and refining of vegetable oils somewhere around the beginning of the last century, trans fatty acids entered our diets. Trans fatty acids are molecularly altered fats resulting from oil refining. They take the place of good fats in the diet, upsetting many important functions in the body as a result (chapter 12). The way to make sure you get enough of the right fats is to avoid all processed foods made with hydrogenated vegetable oil, including margarine, mayonnaise, salad dressings and regular cooking oils. You can get essential fatty acids (good fats) from a whole, natural diet. However, adding a supplement containing essential fatty acids from either fish oils or linseed oil, combined with borage or evening primrose oil can be helpful in general hormone health and for strong bones.

Ipriflavone

Freely available as an over-the-counter supplement, ipriflavone is a synthetic flavinoid derived from the soya isoflavone diadzein. It was first recognised as an effective bone builder in the 1960s in Hungary where it was given as animal feed and was observed to cause an increase in the calcium content of bones in various animals. Ipriflavone is now registered in Europe, Japan and Argentina as a drug for osteoporosis. As it does not occur naturally (except in bee propolis), ipriflavone should technically be classified as a drug. However, due to its relative safety, at present you do not need a prescription for ipriflavone.[122,123]

Unlike other isoflavones, ipriflavone does not possess oestrogenic activity. But because of its similar chemical structure to oestrogen, the body uses it in much the same way to help reduce bone loss. Ipriflavone increases bone density by enhancing the absorption of calcium and phosphorous in the bone. It does this by stimulating the bone-building osteoblasts, while inhibiting the bone breakdown osteoclasts. Ipriflavone is also thought to enhance the secretion of calcitonin (the bone building hormone) and increasing the production of bone matrix proteins.

Caution!

But don't be too quick to self medicate with ipriflavone. A couple of studies have highlighted a potentially dangerous side effect. Participants taking ipriflavone showed a significant drop in lymphocyte (white blood cell) count. As lymphocytes are an important component of the immune system this is not a very desirable side effect. Women who experienced the most severe drop in lymphocyte count took a year or more to recover. If you are tempted to try ipriflavone, it should only be done under medical supervision, and should be avoided by anyone who is already immune compromised, such as people with HIV or those taking drugs to suppress the immune system.[124]

Ideal conditions for *creating* osteoporosis

If you wanted to set out to *create* osteoporosis the following are the ideal conditions and lifestyle choices to make!

• Sedentary occupation with little or no exercise
• Working inside in artificial light with lack of exposure to sunlight
• Using a chemical sun block at first exposure to sun
• Smoking
• Moderate to high consumption of coffee, tea, sugary foods, alcohol, coca cola and chocolate
• A diet high in animal protein, refined carbohydrates and processed fats, such as biscuits, cakes, white pasta and white bread sandwiches
• A low or no fat diet, usually due to a desire to lose weight
• Consuming dairy produce, other than organic, natural yoghurt
• Vitamin and mineral deficiencies caused by crash diets, refined and processed food, too much restaurant food and microwave TV dinners
• Supplements containing large amounts (more than 600 mg) of calcium in the form of carbonate, sulphate or oxide
• Taking diuretics or antibiotics
• Fluoride and chlorine in drinking water

The busy woman's bone protection plan

• Take a regular sunbath whenever you get the chance, building up exposure slowly and without burning, to increase stored vitamin D

• Take regular daily load bearing exercise of 40 minutes minimum such as brisk walking, running on the spot, mini-trampolining, dancing, raquet sports, and running, in the fresh air where possible

• Sleep 8 hours per night

• Eat green, leafy vegetables daily, and choose organically grown produce wherever possible. Add seaweed to your diet in the form of dried flakes to salads and as fresh samphire when in season

• Ensure optimum levels of vitamins and minerals from a wholefood and organic diet and combine with high quality supplements that contain calcium, magnesium, vitamin D, boron, zinc and vitamin K

• Check for low levels of stomach acid with the betaine hydrochloride stomach acid test (page 100)

- Use calcium citrate supplements up to 600 mg per day in place of high dose calcium carbonate and add equivalent amounts of magnesium citrate

- Drink 1 1/2 to 2 litres of mineral or filtered water each day

- Restrict alcohol consumption to no more than 3 - 4 glasses per week. Switch to naturally decaffeinated coffee and drink no more than 2 cups per day. Drink tea very weak, literally dip the tea bag in, count to three and take it out of the cup, or drink herbal varieties

- Substitute dried fruit, high in calcium, magnesium and iron, for chocolate and other sweet foods

- Add unsalted, raw seeds and nuts to your diet daily for their high calcium and magnesium content

- Eat avocados for their essential fatty acids, fibre, vitamin E and vitamin B6 content

- Consume oily fish high in calcium and beneficial oils, such as sardines, salmon, trout, tuna, mackerel three times per week

- Avoid hydrogenated fats and oils. Make salad dressing from cold pressed oils and use reguarlarly. For cooking use naturally saturated oil such as palm oil, coconut oil or butter, or use monunsaturated fats such as olive oil or peanut oil.

PART TWO

HORMONE HEALTH THROUGH OPTIMUM NUTRITION

CHAPTER 11
"LET FOOD BE YOUR MEDICINE"
Hippocrates, the father of medicine

The optimum nutrition approach to women's hormone health is effective, non invasive and does no harm. It also empowers women to take back control of their bodies. Used alongside orthodox medical treatments, e.g. before and after surgery or while taking medication, it provides nutritional support helping the body to detoxify the results of orthodox treatment. At the same time, it provides the building blocks for rebuilding health. As a stand-alone therapy, and when combined with the judicious use of supplements and herbal remedies, the overall effect can be very powerful. Optimum Nutrition works because it creates the biochemical conditions needed for healing.

The busy woman's guide to food

If you already have a good knowledge of food, then you can skip this part. But if you are leading such a busy and stressful life that you have never given much thought to where your food comes from or what processing it might have been through, then you need to understand the basics before you can make healthy choices.

Wholefood (the ultimate goal)

The term 'wholefood' simply means foods which have nothing added and nothing taken away from them. They have not been processed or refined and are as near their natural state as possible. Wholefoods do not contain any artificial additives like flavourings, colourings or preservatives, nor do they contain added fats or sugars.

Wholefoods are important because they are most likely to contain the nutrients your body needs in a form that it can use. For example, when flour is refined to make white bread, it loses most of its 20 vitamins and minerals and almost all of its fibre. Wholemeal bread is made from unrefined flour still containing its fibre, protein, B vitamins, vitamin E and all its minerals.

Chemical 'enhancement'

It is only in the last fifty to one hundred years that man has discovered in the laboratory how to alter food chemically to enhance its keeping, to change its appearance and to exaggerate the sweet, fatty or salty taste. (I am not talking here about salting, drying, pickling and smoking which were more traditional ways of keeping food.) At the same time we are able to farm more intensively with the use of a wide range of chemicals and synthetic fertilisers.

Can we really continue to convince ourselves that this combined cocktail of chemicals has nothing to do with the rising rates of cancers of all kinds, as well as nervous system and autoimmune diseases?

Steering a course through this minefield of refined and processed foods, or healthy foods polluted with toxic fallout from thousands of different chemicals, has become a nightmare for health conscious people.

Back to basics

When choosing what to eat, try and imagine food in its natural state straight from the ground or from the animal or fish. The most processing that it should go through is washing, chopping and, where appropriate, cooking. This is the traditional form of food preparation that has gone on in kitchens for thousands of years. Where possible, buy food that has been grown organically on composted soils and without the use of chemicals before or after picking. This applies to meat and fish as well as to fruit and vegetables.

Food groups

All the foods we eat fall into seven basic food groups (eight if you include water). These are fruit and vegetables, nuts and seeds, grains, pulses, meat and fish, dairy produce, eggs and water. Even processed foods have originally come from these food groups. Identifying the food group to which the components of your next meal belong to is easier if you are consuming whole, unprocessed or refined, natural foods. I have highlighted some power foods further on in this section.

Fruit and vegetables

You can eat both fresh and sun-dried fruit (without the inclusion of food grade mineral oil, glucose or sulphur) 2 – 3 times per day. Fruit makes a good start to the day as it has an alkalising and cleansing effect on the body. Eating fruit regularly also helps with normal weight maintenance and proper elimination of toxins. Both fresh and dried fruit can help you overcome cravings for sweet foods. Some fruits, particularly dried figs, are a good source of calcium and iron.

Vegetables (also includes seaweed high in iodine to nourish the thyroid) are an excellent source of phyto (plant) hormones that help regulate women's hormones

110

and protect against hormone related health problems. They are also an important source of antioxidants that help protect against cancer.

Potatoes are a vegetable and include appreciable amounts of phytohormones. However, because they also contain large amounts of concentrated starch, they are normally categorised with other carbohydrate foods like pasta and rice, and should be eaten in similar (smaller) quantities than other vegetables.

Sugar from sugar beet is a vegetable, while sugar from sugar cane is counted as a grain.

Nuts and seeds

Nuts and seeds are great little nutritional power houses. Choose whole, unblanched, unbroken, unroasted and unsalted nuts and seeds, including almonds, walnuts, hazelnuts, cashews, brazils, pecans, sesame, sunflower seeds, pumpkin seeds and linseeds (flax seed). Peanuts, while not a nut, are a valuable food. Pistachios are often salted and dyed green and therefore best avoided, unless you can find untreated pistachios.

Grains

Grains are from the grass family and include wheat, oats, rye, barley, rice, millet, maize (corn) and buckwheat. All the goodness is in the wholegrain, so ideally you should be eating wholegrain pasta, wholegrain bread and wholegrain rice. Many people initially find the taste of the wholegrain version of their favourite foods a bit heavy going, but it is worth persevering. After a while you realise just how tasteless white refined rice, pasta, bread or pastry really are.

Wholegrains are a valuable source of fibre, vitamins, minerals, essential fatty acids and amino acids (the building blocks of protein). They are also a source of concentrated carbohydrate. The body prefers to manufacture energy from carbohydrates rather than fats. Grains are not the only source of carbohydrates. Fruit and vegetables also provide energy. If you are trying to lose weight you will find it easier if you cut down on concentrated carbohydrates and instead eat fruit and vegetables.

If you rely on convenience foods such as bread, pasta and pastries, you will be restricting your diet and not getting the range of nutrients available in other foods.

111

It is therefore important to obtain energy from a wide range of food groups. Pulses, seeds and nuts also provide valuable carbohydrate energy as well as protein, vitamins, minerals and fibre, although they too are a concentrated source of carbohydrates.

Most people start their day with breakfast cereals which are all grain-based. Some are more refined than others. Muesli is based on raw grains and is a popular break-fast cereal for health-conscious people. Raw grains have one draw back, they contain phytic acid which inhibits the absorption of minerals, especially calcium, iron and zinc, from the intestines. I therefore do not advise eating muesli on a regular daily basis, especially for people suffering from calcium, iron or zinc deficiency, unless it is soaked for a few hours first. Soaking activates the enzymes that help to breaks down the phytates. Because of the binding up of minerals in the intestine I do not recommend giving muesli to growing children.

A note about wheat intolerance

Wheat figures very prominently in the modern western diet. Just think how often you eat bread, breakfast cereals, cakes, biscuits, pizzas, pies, pancakes, crackers, snacks and pasta on a daily basis. Modern strains of wheat contain much higher amounts of gluten (sticky protein that makes bread rise) than wheat grown in our grandparents' day. Gluten is also found in smaller amounts in oats, rye and barley. Some people do not tolerate gluten and experience digestive problems, especially bloating, wind and pain. They do better by avoiding all gluten-containing grains and eating their concentrated carbohydrates in the form of corn, rice, quinoa, millet, buckwheat, and potatoes (not a grain).

Sometimes an allergy to just wheat and not the other grains is due to a group of compounds called lectins. Lectins are also found in peas, beans, lentils and peanuts, all members of the legume family of plants.

Yet other people tolerate no grains at all. They are the 'stone-agers', people whose genes have not adapted to the 'modern' foods like grains introduced when our hunter-gatherer ancestors settled down and started farming a few thousand years ago (chapter 7). Stone-agers do better on fruit, vegetables, seeds and nuts for energy, and they usually do alright with root vegetables like potatoes, carrots and parsnips.

The bottom line is that whole grains, including wheat, are a healthy part of the diet for a lot of people, but not for everyone. If you suspect you might have food intolerance, use the allergy pulse test described in chapter 7.

Pulses

Pulses include lentils and dried beans and peas such as haricot, red kidney, adzuki, borlotti beans and chick peas. They are high in fibre and amino acids as well as vitamins and minerals. They are also low in saturated fat.

Busy women cheat and buy their beans in cans and rinse off the juice they are packed in before using. It saves a lot of time and you don't lose too much in nutritional value.

Because they contain soluble fibre, pulses are particularly useful for women suffering from hormonal symptoms related to blood sugar problems as soluble fibre helps to stabilise blood sugar levels.

Add cooked beans to salads, casseroles, soups and stews, or make hummus or vegetarian burgers from them. Not everyone reacts well to pulses. If you feel unwell, sleepy or have indigestion or wind after eating pulses, avoid them for the time being.

Meat and fish

Meat and fish provide a concentrated source of protein which the body uses for growth, repair and maintenance of every cell and enzyme system in the body. Stone-agers do particularly well obtaining their protein from meat and fish, while others (natural vegetarians) do better healthwise obtaining their protein from vegetarian sources. You don't have to eat meat or fish to have adequate protein. The Seven Day Meal Planner provides small amounts of protein at each meal from both meat/fish and vegetarian sources as part of a balanced diet.

Chicken, pork, beef, lamb, turkey and rabbit are the most commonly eaten meats, and are also the most intensively farmed. Ostrich and game are also available in supermarkets, the latter only in the game season. If you can get organically reared meat then you avoid the dangers of antibiotics, hormones and chemical contamination.

Processed meat and fish, e.g. salami, paté, ham, sausages, bacon, fish spreads, smoked meats and fish, all contain salt, nitrites, saturated fat, often sugar (in the form of dextrose), and E numbers. They should be eaten in moderation only. Ideally, it is better to eat fresh meat and fish that have undergone minimal processing.

Isn't fish full of mercury now?

A lot of fish is farmed intensively nowadays, using regular supplies of antibiotics. A 1999 World Health Organisation report shows that farmed salmon contain less omega-3 fatty acids and around 70% more saturated fat than their wild cousins.[125] Farmed salmon also have dye added to their food to keep their flesh pink (it would normally be grey), and they are routinely fed antibiotics – more per weight than any other livestock, according to a U.S. FDA report.[126]

Ocean going fish do not fare much better. Because of our habit of dumping toxic waste into the ocean, most fish are now contaminated with heavy metals such as mercury. A report from the U.S. Consumer Advisory Center for Food Safety and Applied Nutrition dated March 2001 advises pregnant women to eat no more than 12 oz (340 gm) per week of fish because of the methyl mercury content of ocean going fish. Mercury is particularly high in large fish like swordfish, tuna and shark.[127]

Farmed fish do not have the levels of methyl mercury of wild fish, nor do smaller fish, and it is possible to buy organically farmed fish. Selenium, taken as a supplement of around 200 mcg per day, is antagonistic to mercury, meaning that it helps to escort mercury from the body. My advice is not to give up eating fish, but to choose smaller fish or organically farmed fish and to take appropriate supplementation (chapter 15). You will still feel healthier eating a salmon and vegetable dinner than you will tucking into a packet of biscuits and a chocolate bar. It's worth asking for organic fish at your local fishmonger or supermarket fish counter.

Iron and zinc absorption for vegetarians

While being a vegetarian can be a very healthy way to eat, iron and zinc are better absorbed from meat than they are from vegetables. I have seen a number of vegetarians suffering from iron deficient anaemia and zinc deficiency. Symptoms associated with iron deficiency are fatigue, pale skin, loss of appetite or nausea, sore tongue and getting breathless on light exertion. You can see a zinc deficiency as white spots on the nails. It is also associated with hormone problems, a poor sense of taste or smell, frequent infections, acne or greasy skin, low fertility, pale skin, poor appetite and a tendency to depression. If you are vegetarian and ever find yourself craving a lump of red meat, it could be because your iron or zinc levels are low. If you really cannot stomach the thought of eating meat, but you need extra iron and zinc, try dissolving a teaspoon of black strap molasses in a glass of water and drinking that daily. It doesn't taste too wonderful but molasses is full of iron. Also eat plenty of water cress and parsley as they both contain iron.

Liver used to be a popular source of iron, but unless you can find organic liver, I would not recommend this any more. The liver is the organ of detoxification and concentrates all the pollution to which the animal is exposed.

Milk products

Milk products include milk, yoghurt, cheese, cream, buttermilk, sour cream, butter and ice cream. People who have intolerance problems with cow's milk products often do alright with goat's or ewe's milk, but this is not always the case. I have known a number of women get rid of their sore throats and indigestion when they cut right down on the quantity of cheese they consume. You can live perfectly healthily without milk products (chapter 10).

Eggs

Contrary to popular misconception, eggs do not raise cholesterol levels. Most of the cholesterol in the body is made in the liver as required. Eggs contain lecithin which is essential for correct fat metabolism. Eating the wrong kind of fats, too much refined carbodhydrates and sugar, caffeine consumption and a lack of chromium can interfere with the liver's ability to use fats properly. It is this that can lead to raised cholesterol levels. Eggs are a useful food for those who are not allergic to them as they provide complete protein and a wide range of vitamins and minerals, including iron and sulphur for healthy skin, hair and nails, as well as phytohormones that can influence your own hormones. Buy organic eggs where possible to avoid the concentration of pesticides and environmental contaminants. Organic eggs from free range chickens contain higher levels of lecithin (important for maintaining memory and concentration), than those from factory farmed chickens.

Water

Nature provides us with water to drink. It is the essential 'food' before anything else and every cell in the body needs it to function correctly. The human body is made up of around 70% water.

Carbonated drinks, strong black tea, coffee and alcohol are dehydrating. They upset blood sugar balance, cause a loss of valuable nutrients, including calcium and magnesium, and are a source of toxins, making more work for the liver. Herbal teas can have beneficial properties, as well as being caffeine free. They also add flavour for those who hate drinking plain water.

Most people don't drink enough water. Ideally you need to drink 1 to 2 litres of water per day, more on a hot day. Water can be drunk either hot or cold, still or naturally carbonated, but preferably always filtered or bottled.

Ideal food proportions

The ideal healthy diet should be composed of 70% fresh fruit, vegetables and seeds, with the remaining 30% consisting of meat and fish (for those who eat it), whole grains, pulses (beans and lentils), eggs and nuts. This balances acid and alkaline for general health and for strong bones (chapter 10).

In practical terms, this means eating a good three pieces of fruit, a large mixed salad and a large helping of mixed, steamed vegetables, including dark green leafy vegetables every day. Diagram 5 illustrates what your plate should look like regarding food proportions.

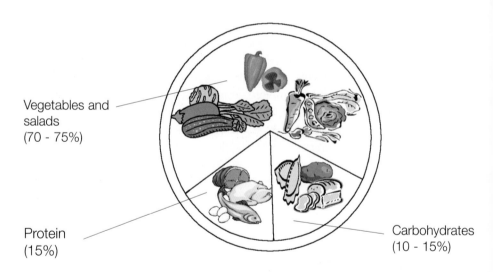

Vegetables and salads (70 - 75%)

Protein (15%)

Carbohydrates (10 - 15%)

Diagram 5. Plate showing ideal food proportions

This way of eating provides a large amount of potassium, needed for a healthy nervous system and to work with magnesium to alleviate muscle cramping. It also provides a lot of useful fibre needed to help excrete toxins and hormones quickly once they have done their job.

Vegetables should be eaten cleaned and raw, or lightly steamed, to retain most of their nutrients and all of their fibre. When vegetables are canned or overcooked, or when fruit is made into desserts with added fat and sugar, they lose much of their nutritional value.

Power foods

All of the following are nutritionally dense foods, that is they contain important amounts of nutrients and essential fatty acids. If you really don't like any of the foods mentioned, please don't feel you have to force yourself to eat them. There is nothing worse than eating for health and vitality and hating every minute of it! The obvious outcome is that you won't stick to your good intentions and you may dismiss all healthy eating as a waste of time. However, if you do like the foods mentioned below, and in the past you have been told to avoid them for weight reasons, then you can rest assured that you can eat them without gaining weight.

Avocados

Avocados are a great source of essential fatty acids, vitamin B6 and zinc. Surprisingly enough, avocados contain a great deal of fibre. The combination of oils and fibre is great for filling you up and maintaining blood sugar levels, which of course means less cravings for sweet foods. The oils in avocados will keep your skin soft and supple and can reduce high cholesterol.

Sun dried fruit

Sun dried fruit, such as apricots, raisins, figs and dates, contain useful quantities of iron, calcium and other vitamins and minerals. They are also great for helping to curb cravings for sweet things. I have known people get over their cravings for chocolate by eating apricots and figs instead! Do make sure you choose sun dried fruit. If apricots are orange, they are not sun dried. They will have been treated with sulphur dioxide to keep their colour. Sun dried apricots are dark brown and treacly in flavour.

But aren't dried fruits high in sugar?

Sun dried fruit contains more concentrated sugar than their fresh counterpart, purely because they have had all the water dried out of them. But the sugar quantity remains the same and is in the form of fructose, which is treated differently by the body than sucrose, the sugar normally used for sweetening.

Dried fruit works well for people with high and low blood sugar levels as they provide a safe and satisfying alternative to sweets, chocolates, cakes and biscuits. I normally recommend eating dried fruit with a piece of fresh fruit and a small handful of seeds and/or nuts to slow down the release of sugar even further.

Seeds and nuts

Like avocados, seeds and nuts deserve a special mention as these foods are most often avoided by people who are worried about gaining weight. This is a mistake as they contain protein, fibre, calcium, magnesium, zinc, chromium, B vitamins, essential fatty acids, and vitamin E (present in the nuts and seeds to protect the oils from rancidity).

Vitamin E works inside your cells in the same way, protecting cell membranes (which are made up largely of fatty acids) from oxidation. This in turn helps to protect against cancer, heart disease and ageing that are triggered by oxidation of fatty acids in the cells. Vitamin E also protects the fats that transport hormones around the body, and raises oestriol levels, making it effective at controlling hot flushes.

Nuts and seeds are a great source of phytohormones and their essential fatty acids are particularly beneficial for balancing hormones. Eat seeds and nuts either as a between-meal snack, or combined with other meals for protein, calcium, magnesium, zinc, B vitamins and essential fatty acids.

Sesame seeds are high in calcium and significant amounts of magnesium which, along with vitamin D, are vital for the absorption of calcium.

Linseeds (flax seed) are a good vegetarian source of omega-3 fatty acids and also contain phytosterols and high amounts of lignans (plant fibres) which can be converted into protective oestrogenic substances. Linseeds have a good reputation for helping to relieve constipation. Grind them or soak and chew them well to get the most benefit from them.

Pumpkin and sunflower seeds are also tasty and full of nutritional goodness, particularly zinc, B vitamins and essential fatty acids.

Of the nuts, choose almonds, cashews, hazelnuts and walnuts to add to breakfast cereals, to a fruit breakfast and to eat as snacks. Brazil nuts are delicious and a good source of selenium but are best eaten in small quantities if you are weight watching as their fat content is the highest of all the nuts.

What about peanuts?

Peanuts, while being a good source of protein and essential fatty acids when eaten raw and straight from their shells, are not nuts and are not such a good source of calcium and magnesium. But providing you do not have any allergies to peanuts, or you do not suffer from candidiasis or other yeast/fungal infections, peanuts are good nutrition.

It is important always to eat nuts and seeds raw and salt free. If they are roasted or salted not only have they lost most of the nutritional benefits, but you will tend to eat more of them. Try eating a packet of raw, unsalted brown skinned almonds and see how soon you have had enough compared with a packet of salted peanuts!

Fermented soya products

Soya, when eaten fermented as a protein source, as it is in the East, provides a very good source of phytoestrogens, particularly isoflavones. The Japanese have no word for 'hot flushes' and the link has been made with their consumption of fermented soya in the form of tofu, miso and tempeh and low rates of breast cancer and menopausal symptoms. In the West we tend to use soya as a substitute for dairy produce rather than as a source of protein. It may not be a good idea to directly swap soya milk for cow's milk as the jury is still out on whether or not too much unfermented soya can abnormally raise oestrogen levels.

As soya is a common allergen and not all women tolerate it very well, I suggest varying the milk substitute you use to include rice, oat, almond and coconut milk in place of regular milk, if you prefer not to consume milk products.

Quinoa

Quinoa has gained in popularity in the west in the past few years, although it has been used as a staple in the high Andes of Peru for millennia. Although used as a grain, quinoa is actually a seed and has all the properties of seeds, i.e. rich in protein, fibre, carbohydrates, vitamins, minerals and essential fatty acids. I was told by a Peruvian gentleman working in Brussels that quinoa is so digestible that they feed it to babies in Peru. A bonus is that it is also gluten 0free, so ideal for people who are gluten sensitive. You can cook whole quinoa like rice and then eat it as an accompaniment in place of rice or pasta, or you can make it into cous cous. Quinoa flakes make good porridge and in health food shops you can buy puffed quinoa and crispy quinoa flakes to be used as breakfast cereals.

Seaweed

Seaweed contains something like forty minerals, including calcium and iodine (important for healthy thyroid function), and is high in phytohormones. It is a very useful addition to everyone's diet. Most seaweed tastes pretty awful to those who are not used to it and usually people try it once and reject it. I have found three forms of seaweed that are actually quite palatable. The first is fresh samphire or salicornia (the same family of seaweed) which is high in valuable oils. They look like green beans all joined together and are available from fish counters in supermarkets when in season. You can rinse samphire and eat it raw in salads, or just plunge it in boiling water for a minute or two, drain and use as you would any other vegetable. Available in health food shops you can also buy Wakama norri flakes that look like powdered parsley. They are great to use in place of salt when cooking fish. For sprinkling on salads, I have discovered *"fisherman's salad"*, which are crispy flakes of norri seaweed.

Because of the nutritional value of seaweed, it really is worth persevering and finding something you like.

Sea salt

Like seaweed, sea salt contains a wide variety of minerals, including iodine, and is a good replacement for regular table salt. Make sure you buy unrefined sea salt. It looks a bit grey in colour and has a less 'salty' taste than regular table salt. Use in small quantities only especially if you are following a low salt diet.

Green tea

Green tea is a tasty alternative to coffee or strong English-style tea. High in phytohormones and antioxidants, green tea helps protect you from free radical damage. Free radicals are electrically unbalanced atoms that cause damage to healthy cells and are a contributory factor to the ageing process, cardiovascular disease, degenerative diseases and cancer.

I recommend drinking green tea very weak, i.e. tea bag in the cup for the count of three and then out again. Drunk this way, green tea gives a very mild lift without over stimulating the adrenals and central nervous system. However, if you need to strictly avoid caffeine in any form, then I am afraid that includes green tea too!

CHAPTER 12
EAT RIGHT FAT, NOT LOW FAT

If there is one area of nutrition that causes more confusion than any other, it's fats. There have been countless books exhorting the benefits of low or no fat diets persuading women to deprive themselves of perfectly natural and healthy foods because they contain fat. In particular is the fear of saturated fats which we are told will make us fat and give us heart disease (actually not true as you will see). This has resulted in women following boring diets consisting of dry chicken breasts, salads with no dressing, and avoiding nuts and avocados, in the belief that this is the only way to lose weight.

Most of the advice given in books about fat misses out one very important factor – the *type* of fat eaten. Not all fats are the same. Some are positively harmful, while others are necessary for good health and a slim figure.

FAQs

"What are the differences among saturated fats, vegetable oils, olive oil, margarine, butter, cheese and the fats contained in bakery products, salad dressings and fatty meat?"

"Why isn't it OK to use sunflower oil for cooking?"

"I only use olive oil for cooking and for salads. That's alright, isn't it?"

"Won't I put on weight if I eat fatty foods like avocados and nuts and use oil on my salads?"

The history

The confusion and misinformation around fats started around a hundred years ago when vegetable oils were first hydrogenated to produce margarine for spreading and baking. Even with the manufacturing process involved, margarine was still a cheaper option than butter for both housewives and the bakery industry. But what manufacturers have been slow to tell us is that the refining and hydrogenation of oils leads to the production of something called *trans fatty acids*, where the molecular structure of oil is changed from a horseshoe shape, or *cis fatty acid*, to a straight line shape, or trans fatty acid. The body knows what to do with cis fatty acids, but is defeated by trans fatty acids, which take the place of cis fatty acids on the receptor sites of cells. In effect, trans fatty acids have an ability to block the conversion of 'good' fats into the components necessary for all the biochemical functions where fatty acids are needed.

The true culprit of heart disease

According to Mary Enig, PhD, to divert public attention away from trans fatty acids, margarine manufacturers focused attention on saturated fat as being the culprit in heart disease, when in fact as early as 1958, a Dr. Ancel Keys was showing that the true culprit was trans fatty acids. This started the "*phoney attack on meat and dairy fats.*"[131]

An expert panel at the U.S. Institute of Medicine issued a detailed review of research into trans fatty acids and came to this conclusion: "*It is recommended that trans fatty acid consumption be as low as possible while consuming a nutritionally adequate diet.*"[128] The U.S. Food and Drug Administration (FDA) is currently in the process of regulating food manufacturers to disclose the trans fatty acid content of their foods on packaging.

The technical data

To clear up the confusion about fats, the different kinds, and their role in health, I have provided a bit of simplified technical data.

Fats fall into two main categories, *saturated* and *unsaturated* fat. Saturation refers to the number of hydrogen atoms attached to a molecule of fat (hence hydrogenated). Saturated fat has all its spare carbon bonds taken up with hydrogen atoms, while unsaturated fat has some carbon atoms joined by double bonds, so there is less room for hydrogen atoms, i.e. unsaturated fat is less hydrogenated.

Unsaturated fats fall into two categories: *monounsaturated* and *polyunsaturated*. Monounsaturated fat, like olive oil, has just one double bond, while polyunsaturated fat, like sunflower oil, has more than one double bond.

Confused?!

In practice, you can tell if a fat is saturated, monounsaturated or polyunsaturated by how solid it goes when refrigerated.

Saturated (hard fat): Butter, cream, lard (animal fat), cheese, coconut oil, palm oil and cocoa butter go hard in the fridge.

Monounsaturated (oil): Olive and peanut oil go a bit cloudy in the fridge.

Polyunsaturated (oil): Nuts, seeds (sunflower, safflower, walnut, sesame, linseed, hazelnut, almond and their oils) and fish oils remain liquid when refrigerated.

To make polyunsaturated oils hard for baking purposes and for margarine, food manufacturers have to add hydrogen atoms, hence the term 'hydrogenated'.

Why we need fat

Fat serves many functions: as 'padding' beneath the skin for warmth and comfort, as a source of energy, in the construction of cell membranes, nerve cells and brain cells, in the manufacture of hormones, for waterproofing skin, and for a healthy heart and strong immune system. Apart from the first two (which use saturated fat), all the other functions are performed by essential fatty acids. They are essential because we cannot manufacture them and we must have them in our diet.

Essential fatty acids (EFAs)

EFAs are important for the production of prostaglandins (PGs), of which there are many types. Prostaglandins are localised hormone-like substances which have an influence on many metabolic functions, including hormone production. Therefore EFAs are particularly important in hormone production and for the transport of hormones around the blood. Many women have found relief from hormone distress by changing the balance of fats in their diet to those that contain essential fatty acids.

Symptoms associated with EFA deficiency[129]

• Dry, rough skin, eczema and psoriasis
• Dry, itchy eyes
• Brittle nails
• Loss of hair or dandruff
• Frequent infections (poor immunity)
• Poor memory and concentration
• Depression and anxiety
• Excessive thirst
• Poor wound healing
• Saliva glands "dry up"
• PMS or breast pain
• Menopausal symptoms

123

- Infertility and miscarriage
- Prostatitis (in men)
- Inflammatory conditions such as arthritis (and achy joints), allergies, auto-immune diseases
- Premature ageing
- Heart disease and high blood pressure
- Hyperactivity (or ADD) in children
- Hypothyroidism and low metabolic rate
- Gastrointestinal problems (particularly leaky gut)
- Blood sugar problems or diabetes
- Tingling sensation in arms and legs
- Motor incoordination

Why evening primrose oil can help with PMS and menopause

EFAs fall into two main groups, or series: linoleic acid (omega-6 series), and alpha-linolenic acid (omega-3 series).

The omega-6 fatty acids are converted to prostaglandins and then to hormones via gamma-linolenic acid (GLA). A lack of omega-6 fatty acids, or the inability to convert them to prostaglandins, can result in any of the signs and symptoms mentioned above. Women who find relief from their symptoms when they take evening primrose oil, borage oil or starflower oil (all good sources of GLA), are either lacking omega-6 fatty acids in their diet, and/or the nutrients needed for the enzyme that converts linoleic acid to GLA, particularly zinc and vitamins B3 and B6. Taking GLA directly cuts out the conversion process from omega-6 fatty acids to GLA.

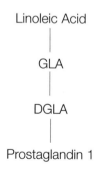

Linoleic Acid

|

GLA

|

DGLA

|

Prostaglandin 1

Diagram 6. Conversion pathway of linoleic acid to prostaglandins

Omega-6 fatty acids are found in all oils made from seeds, particularly sunflower oil, safflower oil and corn oil, providing the oils are cold pressed and unrefined.

124

Linseeds, walnuts, fish oil and the omega-3 fatty acids

Alpha-linolenic acid, an omega-3 fatty acid found in fish oils, walnuts and linseeds, is important for the prevention of heart disease and acts as a natural anti-inflammatory in inflammatory conditions such as arthritis. It is converted into eicosapentaenoic acid (EPA) which can lower cholesterol levels, thin 'sticky' blood, and bring down blood pressure, as well as being important in the production and stability of hormones. It is a good idea to eat oily fish once or twice a week for its EPA content, as well as eating fresh seeds and nuts daily.

Best foods for EFAs

Essential fatty acids are highest in seeds, nuts and the oils made from them. However, they are also found in all vegetables, fruit, grains, pulses, fish and to some extent in organically reared or wild animal fat. Grazing wild animals eat grass and other green plant material which contain essential fatty acids. Be sure to include plenty of green leafy vegetables in your diet too.

Many things can interfere with how the body uses EFAs, including *stress, processed fats and oils, coffee, alcohol and sugar, smoking and processed foods*. Regular daily consumption of alcohol in particular interferes with essential fatty acid metabolism and is a frequent cause of hormone imbalances among women.

Vitamins and minerals are also essential

Certain nutrients are important for the conversion of dietary fatty acids into prostaglandins. These are magnesium, biotin, vitamins B6, B3, C and zinc. Busy women, under stress, eating a diet that is deficient in adequate amounts of vitamins and minerals, can soon find themselves suffering from hormone related problems. Not only are they not eating the right kinds of fats, but they also cannot convert them successfully to prostaglandins and to hormones.

Oil refining

There is one main golden rule to follow when debating what kind of fat to eat: avoid processed fats!

You can easily recognise processed fats. They are the ones that are labelled *"hydrogenated vegetable oil"* on manufactured food products. They are also the ones that will sit in their plastic bottle on the supermarket shelf or in your kitchen cupboard for months or even years and never go off. In her book, *"New Vital Oils"*, Liz Earle[130] gives a list of the heavy refining process that commercial oils go through, involving petrochemicals (hexane), high temperature, bleaching, deodorising and the use of caustic soda to remove all the essential fatty acids, vitamin E, choline, inositol and lecithin, as well as the flavour and smell. In fact all the important ingredients needed for health. While this is very good news for the manufacturers and retailers, it is not good news for you.

Cold pressed oils

It is much better to choose naturally cold pressed oils, such as olive oil and sun-flower oil that have been through a single mechanical pressing at around 80°C, then filtered and bottled. Check labels. If it doesn't say *"cold pressed"*, then it isn't. Keep all cold pressed oils in the fridge (other than olive oil which goes cloudy at cold temperatures).

Cooking and avoiding free radicals

Ideally you should not use fat in cooking and do not cook with cold pressed oils, other than olive or peanut oil, and then only cook at low temperatures. Olive and peanut oil are monounsaturated which means that they are more stable than polyunsaturated fats for cooking. Hazelnut oil and sesame oil are also monoun-saturated and can be lightly heated. This is not the case with sunflower or corn oil.

If you heat the oil to smoking point, throw it away and start again. Heating oils creates free radicals, electrically unbalanced atoms that damage healthy cells and trigger ageing, cardiovascular disease, degenerative diseases and cancer.

The safest fats of all to cook with are the old fashioned animal fats, such as lard and butter, as they are saturated and therefore the most stable at higher temperatures. I still like to add a tiny blob of organic butter when I cook mushrooms because the taste is so good. However, I mostly don't use fat at all, using my conventional oven for most cooking, or I use just a little olive oil if I am cooking food on the hob.

Is it better to eat saturated fat than hydrogenated vegetable oils?

Yes, if the saturated fats come from organically reared animals they contain conju-gated linoleic acid (CLA) which has been shown to help protect against breast cancer and to help maintain lower body fat and increased lean body mass. Palm and coconut oil are also naturally high in saturated fats. So if you enjoy a bit of organic butter on your bread, or coconut milk on your cereal (and you don't have any allergies to either), these make a tasty alternative to regular dairy produce. Cold pressed sunflower oil also contains CLA.

This is not a prescription to eat a lot of fat! If you add oils and fats as shown in the Seven Day Meal Planner (chapter 17), you will be achieving the right proportion of fat in your diet.

Are any margarines alright to use?

It is not a good idea to substitute margarine (even the stuff that is supposed to be good for cholesterol levels) for butter. Generally, margarine is made from hydrogenated vegetable oils and is usually high in trans fatty acids. Check labels carefully. Some products state that they have a high cis fatty acid content (cis fatty acids are the 'good guys', while trans fatty acids are not).

Some products now available from health food stores and major supermarket chains are based solely on naturally saturated plant oils, such as coconut and palm oil, that have not been hydrogenated. They are made from organically grown plants, contain no dairy produce and no chemicals, salt or artificial colouring. They work well in baking and are a reasonable substitute for people who really want to spread a butter look-alike on their bread.

What else to spread on bread

If you don't like butter or have a milk products allergy, then you can use cold pressed olive oil on bread, or spreads made from seeds and nuts. Available in health food shops, these look like peanut butter but are made from sesame or sunflower seeds, hazelnuts, almonds, cashews or a mixture of these. Buy the brands where the oils have risen to the top and have to be stirred back in before using. This shows the least amount of processing. They are delicious and provide a good range of vitamins, minerals, essential fatty acids and protein. Keep seed and nut spreads in the fridge and use them up quickly.

How should I use cold pressed oils?

Throw away all your jars of mayonnaise and salad dressing. They are made from refined oils high in trans fatty acids. Take a look at the recipes (chapter 17) for a cold pressed oil salad dressing that can be used daily to provide the complete set of essential fatty acids for healthy skin, hair, nails and hormones.

As in everything, balance is the key to health. When making salad oil dressings, I find the best combination is to use sunflower and olive oils in equal quantities as the base oils, then add in smaller amounts of linseed oil, pumpkin seed oil and hazelnut or walnut oils for their delicious flavour. Sesame oil gives a different kind of flavour, but is equally delicious. It is particularly good if you are making a creamy dressing with tofu and garlic. Using a variety of oils gives a cross section of mono- and poly- unsaturated fatty acids, as well as providing omegas- 3, 6 and 9 fatty acids.

Most health food stores sell many different kinds of cold pressed oils, usually organic. Keep the polyunsaturated oils in the fridge and the monounsaturated oils in a cool, dark cupboard. Exposure to light, heat and oxygen will shorten the shelf life of cold pressed oils, so do use them regularly and use them up quickly. If you travel a lot, take your cold pressed oil mixture in a vacuum flask and use in place of restaurant dressings.

Liz Earle says that some Italian doctors recommend their patients take a tablespoon of olive oil a day for a healthy heart and soft skin. Add almond oil to your oil base for a sweet taste that is delicious in its own right.

Skin care preparations

If you suffer from dry skin, as well as consuming your oils, you can rub almond and avocado oil into the skin. Olive and coconut oil are also good skin softeners. Most skin preparations, even the most expensive ones, contain petrochemical derivatives. Look out for the words *'parabens'* and *'methylparabens'*, *'petrolatum'*, *'paraffinium'* and *'mineral oil'*, all of which are derived from petrochemicals. It is possible to get face creams and skin care preparations that contain only cold pressed oils such as jojoba, avocado, almond and rose hip, that moisturise and feed the skin. It's worth checking out your health food store and specialist producers.

Addressing the weight issue

Eating fat in whole, natural foods does not cause weight gain. Substitute chocolate bars, alcoholic drinks, coffees, teas, sugary foods and refined carbohydrates with fresh fruit, dried fruits, avocados, seeds and nuts.

Fran's story

Fran was tired of suffering with PMS each month. A single mother of two teenage children and sole wage earner, she couldn't afford to keep taking time off work because of period pains and migraines.

128

Fran also thought she would like to lose a bit of weight as she had put on 9 kg (one and a half stone or around 20 pounds) in the last couple of years, but this wasn't her main concern.

Fran faithfully followed the Seven Day Meal Planner, cutting out stimulants and taking the vitamins, minerals and essential fatty acids recommended to stabilise blood sugar levels. The diet also cut out all trans fatty acids and introduced a generous supply of essential fatty acids.

When I saw her six weeks later, Fran told me she was feeling much better. Her next period had been much less painful. She still had to take a pain killer on the first day, but at least she could go to work and she had more energy.

What really delighted Fran was that when she started eating dried fruit, nuts and seeds, she kicked her daily chocolate habit easily and had lost 6 kg (thirteen and a half pounds, or nearly a stone). Colleagues at work had been quite disparaging about her lunches of avocadoes, tuna and salad, and her mid morning and mid afternoon snacks of fruit, seeds, nuts and raisins.

They told her these food would make her again weight. But when she told them she had lost so much weight and felt heaps better, she noticed that they were surreptitiously bringing in packets of nuts and raisins and eating them when they thought she wasn't looking! She also noticed that they were keeping bottles of water on their desks and drinking more water.

Fran hadn't been sleeping well and had put it down to eating chocolate every evening before bedtime. Now she didn't need chocolate anymore and was sleeping like a baby. No wonder she had more energy!

Three months after starting the programme, Fran had her first completely trouble-free period. "*I didn't even know it was coming. It came on time, with no pain, no irritability and it was lighter with less blood clots than usual.*" She had also lost the 9 kg she had gained before starting the programme.

Weight gain has a number of causes. The obvious is eating too much food for energy output, i.e. if you are not physically active and you eat too much you will lay down fat. A low metabolic rate caused by a sluggish thyroid can make it difficult for women to lose weight. Eating too many sugar promoting foods increases insulin production. One of insulin's jobs is to turn excess sugar in the blood into fat. In the next section on blood sugar control, you will see how to control cravings, eat less and develop a taste for foods that maintain even blood sugar, energy and happy hormones.

CHAPTER 13
BLOOD SUGAR CONTROL

Of all the aspects of diet that most affect hormone function and health, blood sugar control is probably the most important. It is the first thing I check when someone tells me they suffer from PMS or night sweats because erratic blood sugar contributes to both.

The energy cycle

All energy comes from sugar in the form of glucose circulating round the body. The glucose is a breakdown product of the carbohydrates in food, e.g. potatoes, rice, pasta, bread, cereals, seeds, nuts, pulses, sugar, cakes, biscuits, croissants, pizzas, fruit and vegetables.

When food is whole and unrefined, for example wholemeal bread, the carbohydrates are broken down more slowly as they have to be extracted from their fibrous coating. Once released, the carbohydrates are then turned into glucose in the liver and released slowly into the blood on an 'as needed basis'. If the carbohydrates are attached to a fat, i.e. butter or seed spread on bread, this slows down the breakdown and absorption of the glucose even further.

Quick sugar release

On the other hand a croissant contains refined, white flour and white, refined sugar, which is rapidly released into the blood, by-passing the liver , even though it also contains some fat (usually hydrogenated). Blood sugar levels then rise quickly, usually too quickly and too high for safety. To adjust the levels and bring them back into the normal range, the pancreas releases insulin to 'mop up' the excess sugar. One of insulin's jobs is to turn excess sugar into fat if there is no more room in the usual storage depots (muscles and liver). High insulin levels can therefore lead to weight gain and obesity.

Regular high levels of insulin due to high levels of glucose in the blood can also feed cancer cells as they use glucose for fuel, according to Otto Warburg, PhD, 1931 Nobel laureate in medicine. His paper revealing this research was first published in 1956. So the information about the connection between sugar consumption and cancer has been around for a long time![132]

People consuming sugar or refined carbohydrates on a regular basis are putting their pancreas and insulin production under a lot of strain and, in susceptible individuals, the end result may be diabetes.

The problem is compounded with the consumption of foods that, while not sugar in themselves, promote the release of sugar in the blood. These are caffeine - found in coffee, tea, cola drinks and cocoa (including chocolate and drinking chocolate) - alcohol and tobacco. Highly salted snacks also cause a rise in blood sugar levels.

Lack of nutrients

Refined foods are devoid of the nutrients needed to feed the enzyme systems that govern blood sugar control, particularly the B vitamins, zinc, chromium and manganese. Eventually, the sugar regulating mechanisms start to malfunction. At best people find themselves experiencing energy highs and lows, and eventually not even the highs.

We're all sensitised to sugar

Because all people living in the developed countries of the world have been sensitised to sugar over the last 150 to 200 years, it is likely that the majority of people suffer from some degree of *disglycaemia*. This is the term used to describe erratically fluctuating blood sugar levels with bouts of *hyperglycaemia* (high blood sugar) and *hypoglycaemia* (low blood sugar). Rapid and sharp swings in blood sugar levels can effect brain chemistry, leading to the typical emotional and mental symptoms associated with PMS and the menopause.

While I have only ever experienced the symptoms of PMS on four or five occasions, I suffered with quite bad disglycaemia when I was younger. When my blood sugar levels got too high, I felt hyper, a bit dizzy, spaced out and found myself stumbling over words as I lost slight speech coordination. When they dropped too low, I found it hard remembering things and keeping thoughts in my head from one minute to the next. I felt so tired that all I wanted to do was fall asleep. I got irritable and anxious and felt very empty and needed to eat, even though I knew I wasn't really hungry.

On a sugar-free, low carbohydrate diet, avoiding caffeine and chocolate, my energy levels are constant and my moods are stable. If bad habits, usually caffeine or chocolate even in very small amounts, start to creep in on a regular daily basis, then I can feel my blood sugar start to swing up and down again.

The many women who have regained blood sugar control say they can feel the effects almost instantly once they have changed their eating habits. Whereas before they had no idea that their daily cups of coffee, chocolate bars and white bread sandwiches were having any effect, now they know that it does make a difference to how well they feel.

Insulin resistance, polycystic ovaries and diabetes

Regular high sugar consumption can over time lead to insulin resistance. This is where the pancreas continues to produce insulin in response to the high blood sugar levels, but the body is no longer able to respond to it and blood sugar levels stay too high.

Polycystic ovaries is a condition caused by an increase in circulating androgens and oestrogens, the latter due to increased conversion of androgens to oestrogens, and low levels of DHEA. Women with polycystic ovaries are usually found to have insulin resistance. They also have some degree of obesity and suffer from symptoms associated with hormone imbalance in favour of male hormones, notably hirsuitism (increase in facial and body hair), amenorrhea (no periods) and enlarged ovaries with multiple small cysts. Polycystic ovarian disease is a frequent cause of infertility. While there is no evidence to suggest that sugar may be a direct cause of this condition, raised insulin levels and obesity are certainly contributing factors.[133]

Insulin resistance is a high risk factor in the development of diabetes. Avoiding sugar will help lower insulin which is normally secreted in response to sugar promoting foods and drinks.

Helen's story

Helen was a young women in her late twenties who came to see me for weight problems. At 165 cm (5' 5") she weighed 89 kg (around 14 stone or 200 pounds). Her goal was to lose about twenty kilos but no matter what she did, she just could not lose weight. She told me that she was also suffering from polycystic ovaries, experienced vaginal thrush before each period, and her periods were very heavy and painful. Blood test results showed that she had low levels of DHEA and progesterone, and raised levels of oestrogen and testosterone. Her blood sugar levels were also high. Further tests confirmed candida as a contributing factor to her health problems.

I persuaded Helen to give up her four to five cups of coffee and one cup of tea per day, as well as her daily chocolate habit, all of which were stimulating raised insulin levels. Getting her to cut down on her pack of cigarettes per day presented a bit more of a challenge. I advised Helen to follow my anti-candida nutrition programme, gradually cutting down on all her insulin promoting foods and substituting more fresh fruit, vegetables, fish, chicken, seeds, nuts and quinoa. She also gave up dairy produce and foods containing wheat. I recommended supplements that included a herbal anti-fungal based on pau d'arco and garlic, a multi vitamin and mineral complex, essential fatty acids, chromium, magnesium, vitamin E and hydroxy citric acid (HCA to help the body convert carbohydrates into glucose energy rather than fat). Her doctor prescribed DHEA and natural progesterone.

Just one month after coming to see me, Helen reported having a lighter, less painful period that was not preceded by a thrush attack. She had also lost four kilos (about nine pounds or just over half a stone) in weight and was feeling more energetic. Within three months, Helen's blood sugar levels were back within normal range, although her hormones were taking longer to get back in balance. She had also lost ten kilos (twenty two and a half pounds or over one and a half stone) and her periods continued to be light and much less painful. Helen moved away after that and I didn't get to follow her progress, but with a good doctor to monitor her hormone balance and good nutritional support, Helen had a very good chance of regaining her full hormone health within the year.

The glycaemic table

"I've heard that eating carrots and rice causes a rise in blood sugar – how can that be true?" Sue P, Administrator

In the last few years a lot of research has been done on the glycaemic (blood sugar) effect of foods. The Glycemic Research Institute in Washington DC has produced the Glycaemic Index, a list of foods that unfavourably alter blood sugar levels and contribute to the ever growing problem of obesity in the States.[134] The Institute has scored foods as having a high or low effect on blood sugar. Some of the foods scoring high are the obvious ones like sugar, Mars bars, fructose and refined breakfast cereals. What is surprising, however, is that some apparently healthy foods also score high on the glycaemic table. For example, wholemeal bread has a higher score than white spaghetti (which is made from refined flour), cooked carrots have a higher score than a Mars bar, and new potatoes and raisins have a higher score than sugar !

Adding fat and protein

Blood sugar is not quite as simplistic as the Glycaemic Index might at first indicate. Fat and protein eaten at the same time as carbohydrate slow down the rate of absorption and release of glucose. One of the reasons that a chocolate bar will have a lower score than cooked carrots is because of the fat content. People rarely eat cooked carrots or potato on their own. If you eat potato and carrots with oil or butter, beans, meat, fish, eggs, or tofu (all of which have a low glycaemic score), the rate of glucose release is slowed down.

I often suggest that people eat dried fruits to satisfy cravings as they contain concentrated fructose sugar, fibre, vitamins and minerals. Dried fruit has a high glycaemic score, yet if it is eaten with a few nuts and seeds, e.g. almonds or sunflower seeds, both of which contain oils and protein, the effect of the sugar in the fruit is much more gentle and long lasting. In any case, fructose is treated differently by the body than white sugar. It doesn't normally empty straight into the blood from the intestines, but goes to the liver first where it is broken down and released when blood sugar levels fall.

The Glycaemic Index can be very confusing for people who want to lose weight and still eat healthy food. The most important aspect of healthy weight loss is the elimination of refined carbohydrate, sugar, caffeine, alcohol, chocolate and salty snacks to avoid the secretion of insulin. If a woman suffers from low thyroid function or other form of endocrine disruption, she may find it difficult to lose weight even on a low carbohydrate diet. But normally people lose weight when they combine regular exercise with a diet containing unrefined foods, including potatoes, carrots, dried fruit and bananas – all the high scoring foods. The average weight loss following the Seven Day Meal Planner is 4 kg (9 lbs) in the first month, 2 kg (4.5 lbs) in the second month, and 1 kg (2.25 lbs) per month thereafter until the desired weight has been reached. Everyone is different of course, and some people lose a lot more initially, and others lose less. But they nearly all lose consistently.

Those who put the weight back on after losing it do so when they reintroduce alcohol, coffee, sugar, chocolate and desserts back into their diet, confirming that these are worse culprits for weight gain than dried fruit or baked potato.

Food sensitivity and hypoglycaemia

Sensitivity to certain foods can cause disruption in blood sugar control, even healthy foods, leading to something called 'reactive hypoglycaemia' when blood sugar levels drop in response to a food trigger. The most common food groups known to cause intolerance are wheat and dairy products, followed by oats and rye, eggs, oranges, soya, nuts, seeds and the nightshade family (potatoes, tomatoes, bell peppers and aubergines).

However, just about any food can cause sensitivity in some people, and it can be different foods for different people – it's very much an individual reaction. This is regardless of the fact that these are normally healthy foods. If someone has become sensitive to say wheat, then eating a slice of bread can play havoc with blood sugar control. Removing sensitive items from the diet leads to more energy, a less foggy brain and more emotional and mental stability.

Cathleen's story

Cathleen was a young woman who had not had any periods for about three years (amenorrhea). She had a history of mild anorexia, which was now under control, although she still had some anxiety around food. She was slightly underweight but her doctor had declared her overall body fat sufficient to have periods. There was nothing organically wrong with her. As well as amenorrhoea, Cathleen also suffered from hair loss, dry skin and hair, numerous allergies manifesting as hayfever, asthma and eczema, and muscle tremors, particularly shakes in her hands. She also often felt spaced out, anxious, depressed and lacking in energy.

A low allergy diet with supplements containing Vitex Agnus Castus, zinc and magnesium brought her periods back. Cathleen also had more energy, less anxiety and depression, and she had lost that 'spacey' sensation. Wheat didn't seem to be a problem for Cathleen, and it wasn't until she stopped eating rice, a less common allergen in the west, that her muscle tremors subsided.

Normal blood sugar control

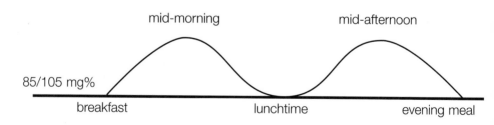

Diagram 8. Normal blood sugar

Normal functioning blood sugar control starts off in the morning with a fasting rate of around 85 mg of sugar per litre of blood, expressed as mg%. After eating the first meal of the day, blood sugar levels should rise evenly over the next couple of hours, and gradually start to fall so that by the next meal 4 to 5 hours later, hunger and the need to eat has set in. The same process is repeated after the midday meal until the evening meal 5 to 6 hours later. Diagram 8 shows you what normal blood sugar control should look like.

With blood sugar levels like this, you feel calm, energetic and have a sense of well being throughout the day. You also sleep well and are less likely to have problems with your hormones when you have balanced blood sugar.

Disglycaemia

Because of less than adequate diets and stressful lifestyles, blood sugar levels are much more likely to look like this:

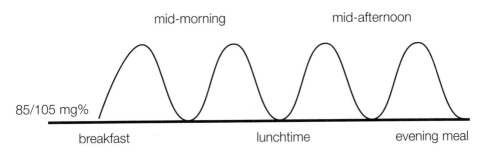

Diagram 9. Disglycaemia

If your blood sugar levels are doing this you will suffer from erratic energy, sometimes feeling full of beans, and then suddenly feeling very tired, listless and lacking energy. Eventually, you won't even have the highs, but will suffer from a perpetual 'dragging round a lead weight' kind of fatigue that leaves you feeling drained.

This level of fatigue is a source of physical stress and causes your adrenals to be in a constant state of alert, using up cortisol (stress hormone) faster than normal. As cortisol competes with progesterone, from which it is made, over time you will produce insufficient amounts of progesterone to balance oestrogen. If oestrogen becomes more dominant, you will suffer much more from hormone fluctuations and the symptoms of PMS and menopause.

Hypoglycaemia

Hypoglycaemia just means low blood sugar. The following symptoms are a clue that you may be suffering from bouts of hypoglycaemia :

- Extreme hunger, light headedness and dizziness
- Headaches, nausea and muscle tremors
- Irritability, mood swings, aggressive or tearful outbursts and extreme impatience
- Nervousness, anxiety and depression
- Loss of memory and lack of concentration
- Lethargy, drowsiness, fatigue and lack of energy
- Sweating, particularly night sweats
- Heart palpitations
- Pallor (growing pale)
- Thirst
- Restless sleep and bad dreams
- Low blood pressure and feeling cold

Not everyone has all of the above symptoms and individuals react differently. One person may yawn and feel sleepy, while another may become hungry and grow pale. Generally speaking, the lower the blood sugar, the lower is the blood pressure and the lower the body temperature. It is not uncommon for women with night sweats to also experience bad dreams and restless sleep or insomnia. Waking in the morning with a dull headache can also be a sign of low blood sugar.

Many of the symptoms of poor blood sugar control are the same as those of PMS and the menopause. In fact when I go through the symptoms associated with dis-glycaemia and hypoglycaemia, most of my clients remark that they are the same as their PMS!

Night sweats and hot flushes that cause extreme sweating, while normally associated with declining oestrogen levels in menopausal women, are very closely related to fluctuating blood sugar levels caused by too much sugar primarily, but also caffeine and alcohol. When women restore their blood sugar balance by removing sugar, caffeine and alcohol from their diet, their heavy sweating and night sweats soon start to disappear.

Normal blood test results

"My blood test says that my blood sugar is normal, but I feel terrible and my symptoms are the same as those for hypoglycaemia." Kate M, Human Resources Manager

Many women have obvious symptoms of disglycaemia yet they have normal blood sugar test results. According to Ray C. Wunderlich, MD, in his book *'Sugar and your Health'*, this is due to lowered levels of glucose in the brain, even when they are adequate in the blood.[135] The brain perceives a drop in blood sugar, where none exists. This implies that blood tests are not necessarily the most effective way of telling if you are suffering from disglycaemia. The symptoms listed above are a pretty good indication of whether or not someone is suffering from poor blood sugar control.

Dr. Wunderlich explains that because everyone is different, people have individual reactions to sugar and the way they metabolise it. This is reflected in blood test results. A *'normal'* blood sugar level may be different from one person to the next. What is optimal for one, may not be optimal for another. Usually levels that fall below 60 or 70 mg% are considered low. But for the person whose normal level is, say, 115 mg%, a drop to 85mg% could represent low blood sugar for them.

As a guide, 85 mg% is considered a normal fasting rate, i.e. first thing in the morning before breakfast. A blood fasting rate of 70mg% indicate low blood sugar. Blood fasting rates of 100 to 110mg% would indicate a need to reduce sugar and refined carbohydrates.

If you have a blood test done after eating, levels should not exceed 160 – 170 mg% after one hour, although some authorities recognise 200 mg% as the upper limit.

Your doctor is the best person to assess whether or not you have dangerously high or low blood sugar levels. If your red blood cells have become sugar-coated (*glycosilated haemoglobin*), as they can do in high blood sugar, your doctor will certainly take action to reduce blood sugar. When some doctors have referred their patients to me with glycosilated heomoglobin, I usually find that blood sugar levels respond within three months to the optimum nutrition nutrition approach.

If you have normal blood test results, but still suffer from many of the symptoms associated with blood sugar fluctuations, you will benefit from the nutritional recommendations for regulating blood sugar.

The 2 - 4 o'clock blues

The phenomenon of the mid-morning and mid-afternoon blues, or energy slump, when you feel drowsy and reach for a coffee, tea, hot chocolate, cola drink or chocolate bar to 'pick-me-up', is well known to many people. Diagram 9 shows that a mid-morning and mid-afternoon slump in energy are pretty normal for people suffering from blood sugar fluctuations. But even in people with normal blood sugar control, it is quite normal to feel a bit sleepy between 2 p.m. and 4 p.m. as this is a natural down-time in our circadian (24 hour daily) rhythms.

Power naps

Some years ago I attended a fatigue conference in Paris being given by the NASA Ames 'Z' team.[136] The team had spent much time investigating the human need for sleep and the role of sleep deprivation in human error and accidents. Their research led them to believe that the majority of people in industrialised countries are running on a sleep deficit and it is this lack of sleep that leads to so many accidents and mistakes caused by human error. The 'Z' team's investigations found that sleep deprivation was the cause of airline crashes, driving accidents, nuclear reactor leaks (Chernobyl), and to less crucial but still annoying mistakes such as poor business decisions or forgetting an important appointment.

The 'Z' team discovered that we are designed to have around eight hours sleep a night with an afternoon siesta of about an hour. Mid-afternoon is when energy levels take a natural dip. As most people in a working situation are unable to take time off for an hour's sleep in the middle of the afternoon, the 'Z' Team recommend a ten to twenty minute "*power nap*" to recuperate sagging energy. If you are able to put a 'keep out' sign on your office door for ten to twenty minutes after lunch, your organisation will benefit from a more alert employee in the afternoon. Of course this won't work if you are in an open plan office or if you have a workaholic boss! However, ten minutes of quiet meditation at your desk, just switching off from everything around you, can also be beneficial as it gives the brain a rest.

Instead of working people into the ground, it should be common practice for companies to insist on breaks mid-morning, mid-afternoon and lunchtime. I once worked for an multi-national company and was impressed with their policy that employees should take a break from their desk for 15 - 20 minutes half way through the morning and afternoon, and that they should leave their desk for a minimum of 30 minutes at lunchtime. Employees were not allowed to eat and drink at their desk through these breaks. The company provided an excellent canteen with plenty of healthy choices. A very civilised way of safeguarding the health of an organisation's most important asset - its people!

Nutritional stressors and blood sugar control

Nutritional stressors are stimulating substances used on a daily basis to "*keep me going*", "*give me energy*", "*calm me down*" and "*help me to wake up in the morning*". Many women are dependent on them but because they are so commonly used they are not regarded as a source of concern.

Here they are:

• Caffeine found in coffee, tea, chocolate and cocoa products, and cola drinks
• Alcohol
• Sugar (and sugary foods/drinks)
• Tobacco and smoking
• Salt (and highly salted foods and snacks)

Most people imagine they couldn't possibly get through a single day without at least one of these!

Nutritional stressors deplete the body of the vital nutrients needed to produce and regulate hormones, namely magnesium, zinc, B vitamins, especially B3 and B6, manganese, chromium and vitamin C. They also have a direct biochemical effect on hormone balance, leading to symptoms associated with PMS and the menopause.

Caffeine

Caffeine, found in tea, coffee and cocoa products, including chocolate, is a useful substance for energy when you really need it, for example driving on a long journey or when you have to work late to meet a deadline, but it has many downsides. Caffeine 'leaches' valuable water soluble B vitamins, as well as reducing zinc, iron and magnesium levels, all of which are needed for energy and mental stability. Overuse of caffeine (and even one cup of coffee or tea a day can be too much for sensitive people) upsets the central nervous system and can cause jittery nerves, anxiety, depression and insomnia.

Caffeine is detoxified in the liver. Some people are very good caffeine detoxifiers and others are not. As one of the world's worst caffeine detoxifiers, I get a buzz even on a weak decaffeinated coffee (there's still about 1% caffeine left in a decaf coffee). Drinking regular coffee is like putting poison in my body. The caffeine is still there whizzing around my system 24 hours later. My sleep is disturbed and my blood sugar levels get out of balance. I get dark circles under my eyes when I consume anything with caffeine, including chocolate - a sure sign that I am sensitive to it. Many women report feeling less anxious, depressed and lethargic and having *more* energy when they give up caffeine.

On the other hand, there are people who are great caffeine detoxifiers. They are the ones who can drink several cups of coffee a day, feel good, look good, have a calm energy and sleep well. This doesn't mean to say that the caffeine is not having any harmful effects, just that their liver's deal with it more effectively.

Sugar and sugary foods

The white sugar used freely by the food manufacturers in everything savoury as well as sweet, is usually based on sugar beet or sugar cane, and has no part to play in a healthy, wholefood diet. White sugar is what is left after the original whole product (cane or beet) has been through several refining processes removing all the vitamins, minerals, protein and fibre.

Sugar has a profound effect on the body's ability to regulate blood sugar levels, which need to remain reasonably stable if your brain is to function normally. It has an almost drug-like action on body chemistry in that it can become quite addictive for some people, as well as altering mood and behaviour. Regular sugar consumers often feel irritable, tense, anxious, depressed or even aggressive for no apparent reason. Does this sound like anyone you know? Take a look round at your colleagues, friends and loved ones, and notice the amount of sugar, caffeine and alcohol they are consuming. You will soon realise that their sudden outbursts, aggressive behaviour, emotional instability and irritability may be symptoms of disglycaemia!

Over-consumption of sugar is like putting jet fuel into your car and will eventually damage the pancreas' ability to control blood sugar levels successfully. Eating foods made with refined sugar robs you of many valuable nutrients which are needed for their metabolism, in particular chromium, manganese, B vitamins, zinc and magnesium. Sugar contains none of these, so they have to come from somewhere. Unless you are taking supplements you will soon become depleted. The rising rate of diabetes in the West is in no small part due to sugar consumption and a lack of chromium and manganese in our diets. Besides erratic blood sugar control, another symptom of manganese deficiency is joint problems as manganese is required for cartilage and bone production.

Because chromium and manganese are important for helping to control blood sugar levels and for curbing cravings, I recommend chromium combined with manganese as part of a comprehensive nutrition programme to successfully counteract the cravings associated with PMS.

Check labels, you may be surprised at just how much sugar is being added to even savoury foods. Other words that mean sugar are *monosaccharide, polysaccharides, date sugar, syrup, cane sugar, glycogen, mannitol, sorbitol, aspartame*, and all words ending in *–ose*, e.g. *dextrose, sucrose, fructose, maltose, lactose, galactose*.

Alcohol

"But I thought red wine was meant to be good for you!"

Some research was done a few years ago to show that drinking red wine helped prevent heart disease. This research was done on men, not women. When they media reported these findings, they did not draw attention to the fact that the substances in wine that protect the heart, i.e. anthocyanadines, are present in the skins of red grapes from which the wine is made. Anthocyanidins are powerful antioxidants and are important for protecting against degenerative diseases and ageing. You don't need to drink red wine for anthocyanidins. You can get all the protection you need from eating a bunch of red grapes or drinking red grape juice (without the alcohol!). Anthocyanidins are also found in bilberries and good quality supplements often contain bilberry extract.

Despite the research that says it's beneficial to drink one or two glasses of red wine every day, the American Cancer Society (ACS) warns that alcohol consumption may in fact increase the risk for breast cancer in women.[137] Alcohol changes a woman's hormones by potentiating the effect of oestrogen (making it stronger) and by interfering with essential fatty acid metabolism. Alcohol may also block the liver's ability to process oestradiol. As far as your liver is concerned, alcohol is just one more toxin to be processed - no matter how expensive the wine, beer or spirit you have drunk.

All alcohol consumption causes a depletion of zinc, magnesium and B vitamins, which can increase feelings of fatigue, stress and brain 'fog'. It also interferes with essential fatty acid metabolism, leading to symptoms of breast pain and tenderness.

Busy and stressed out women often reach for a glass or two of wine to help them relax at the end of a hectic day. But the ACS research suggests that less than one drink a day on average can increase a postmenopausal woman's chances of dying from breast cancer by 30% compared to women who do not consume alcohol.[138] Premenopausal women also have an increased risk of breast cancer but so far no

143

safe limit has been set. (Setting a safe limit is always difficult partly because each individual is different in their ability to detoxify alcohol.)

The real issue seems to be regular, daily consumption of alcohol, whether wine, beer or spirits, rather than the odd drink now and again. Women going through the menopause often notice that their tolerance for alcohol decreases and some just give up drinking altogether because it stops being a pleasant experience.

When it comes to peaceful night's sleep, the NASA Ames 'Z' Team report that alcohol disturbs sleep patterns and leads to a poor night's sleep and causes sleep apnoea. They advise against drinking before going to bed as a means of getting to sleep because, while you may drop off more quickly with a drink, you can have problems staying asleep.

With alcohol-induced sleep apnoea, you will be waking many times during the night, usually without even knowing it. I have one or two clients who have reported feeling exhausted all the time. When they have been to a sleep clinic for investigation, they discover that they have sleep apnoea, never sleep deeply and are waking up sometimes more than one hundred times per hour, without being aware of it!

If you are stressed out, suffering from hormone related health problems, PMS, breast tenderness, menopausal sweats, hot flushes and insomnia, you will feel less stressed, sleep better and have happier hormones if you limit alcohol consumption to no more than two to four glasses per week *maxiumum*. Stay in tune with your body, if even that amount of alcohol feels as though it may be affecting you, try giving up for a while and see if you feel any better.

"I decided to stop my evening couple of glasses of wine on your suggestion, just as an experiment. Do you think it's a coincidence that now, after five days of no wine, my brain feels less fogged up and I can think more clearly? I also feel less tired and stressed and have the impression that I am sleeping more deeply." Mary G, Lawyer

Salt and salty snacks

High salt consumption leads to an imbalance in potassium in the body. Potassium is very important for your nervous system and in your muscles. Signs of potassium deficiency are muscle weakness, spasms and cramps, rapid heartbeat, high blood pressure, listlessness and feelings of apprehension.

Magnesium is important for keeping potassium in the cells. If you are a high alcohol or coffee consumer, as well as eating large amounts of salty foods, you can soon become potassium deficient. Painful periods and cramping muscles are usually a good indication of potassium and magnesium deficiency.

Unrefined sea salt can actually add valuable minerals to food, as well as a taste of the sea. Don't go overboard, but using a pinch here and there is far better than using regular table salt.

Smoking

The toxins in cigarettes affect every part of your body as they pass into the bloodstream and circulate everywhere. Cigarettes don't just increase your risk of lung cancer – if that were the case then it might be worth taking the risk for a determined smoker, as all smokers don't end up with lung cancer.

The poisons circulating in your blood from smoking undermine your immune system, your liver (which has to detoxify them) and your endocrine system, all of which can make you more prone to other forms of cancer, including hormone related cancers. Taking the Pill and smoking increases the risk of death from thrombosis.

Nicotine is highly addictive, even more addictive than cocaine. It picks you up when you feel down, makes you relaxed when you are stressed, kills appetite if you want to lose weight, and alters brain chemistry so that you can't do without it. Smoking causes the skin to age more quickly than a non-smoker's and robs smokers of zinc, calcium, magnesium, B vitamins and vitamin C. It makes clothes, hair and home smell (disgusting to non-smokers) and passive smoke may give someone else an asthma attack or even cancer. It will certainly make someone's evening out an unpleasant experience, even if the smoker is having a good time.

If you smoke, seek help to give it up. Some women have succeeded in giving up using aural acupuncture (needles in the outside of the ear) and hypnotherapy. Revising your diet, rebalancing blood sugar, taking supplements, including l-glutamine, and taking more exercise will put you in a much better position health wise to give up smoking and to resist starting again.

Sometimes fear is the motivation required to giving up smoking. One of my clients who smoked about twenty a day for years, noticed a sore on her tongue. Researching the internet convinced her that the sore could be tongue cancer. She stopped smoking immediately! As it turned out, the sore wasn't cancer, but she had had enough of a shock to remain a non-smoker ever since!

Controlling the nutritional stressors habit

If you suffer from breast tenderness, mood swings or depression, cutting out nutritional stressors for a month or two can make a huge difference. Cutting down or giving up nutritional stressors is hard. But once you have got them out of your system, you can use them for the stimulants they really are, on an occasional or 'as-needed' basis. When you do decide to indulge in, say, a cup of coffee or piece of chocolate, you will find you get much more of a lift on a lot less stimulant. Be sure to always indulge in the very best quality 'abusive substance', i.e. no instant coffee, cheap plonk or chocolate containing hydrogenated vegetable oils and a list of 'E' numbers. Plain (dark) Belgian chocolate contains cocoa solids, cocoa butter and sugar. Actually, a relatively 'natural' product! Make your nutritional stressor a treat to be savoured and not an every day occurrence that hardly gets noticed.

Isn't a headache on giving up coffee a sign you shouldn't give it up?

"I had a splitting headache the first two days of not drinking coffee! And when I took the magnesium you recommended it made falling asleep much easier. I'm now actually getting a good night's sleep. I'm impressed!" Sheila H, Secretary

A lot of women who cut out nutritional stressors experience a withdrawal headache for up to 48 hours. Some experience severe withdrawal symptoms.

"I nearly rang you in the middle of the night, I felt so bad and thought I must have caught a virus or something. My whole body ached, my head throbbed, I felt sick and I couldn't lie down in bed I felt so achy and restless. Anyway, I took a paracetamol and was able to get some sleep. The next day I felt weak and still had a headache but it wasn't quite so bad. After three days, that all went away, but it wasn't until two weeks after no nutritional stressors, that I suddenly woke up before the alarm and felt full of the joys of spring. Amazing! Haven't felt like this since I was about six! " Josephine M, Translator

You can choose to go 'cold turkey' and just cut out all your stimulants, or you can phase them out gradually over a couple of weeks. Switch to naturally decaffeinated coffee (decaffeinated with carbon dioxide and water) as an interim measure. Try also herbal teas, weak green china tea or jasmine tea, rooibos tea (red leaf, caffeine-free tea from S. Africa), cereal based coffee substitutes, chicory and fruit juices. Bear in mind that even green tea and decaffeinated coffee contain small amounts of caffeine. Above all, plain filtered or bottled water is the essential liquid to life and health.

Strategy for good blood sugar control

There is a way to ensure even blood sugar levels all day long, giving more energy and better concentration. It involves eating regular meals with snacks of fresh fruit and nuts or seeds between meals. The secret is not to wait until you are keeling over with hunger, cravings and low energy. A little and often is preferable.

Breakfast - or instead of breakfast

Start the day with breakfast, no matter how light, and no tea or coffee to 'get you going'. Breakfast can contain a choice or mixture of fruit, whole grain cereals, some protein in the form of nuts and seeds, live yoghurt or eggs. Some people find cereals make them more sleepy in the mornings. This especially applies if you have an intolerance to cereals or if you have a particularly poor blood sugar control. Nuts and seeds are a good source of energy, vitamins, minerals and essential fatty acids. You could try live yoghurt with chopped bananas and seeds. For big appetites you could have avocados or a protein breakfast based on eggs, cold meat or fish.

If you really can't stomach the thought of breakfast, have a glass of freshly squeezed fruit juice and a cup of hot water, with or without a slice of lemon, or herbal tea. Many women have discovered the joys of drinking hot water – honestly! – even those who told me, "No way!" to begin with.

A very light start to the morning is a fruit shake made with soft fruit of choice (banana, strawberries, raspberries, peaches, blackberries – whatever is in season) liquidised with mineral water, cashew nuts and almonds, and a mixture of sunflower, pumpkin seeds and linseed. Drink immediately.

If you are a non-breakfast person, just remember to take something with you for later such as a wholemeal sandwich or rice cakes spread with seed or nut spreads, fresh fruit, dried fruit, seeds and nuts. If you are not prepared, you will experience a sudden dip in blood sugar about half way through the morning and find yourself rushing to the coffee machine or buying a chocolate bar or croissant to fill the gap.

Regular meals

Make sure you eat every four hours at the very least, with snacks of fresh and dried fruit, seeds, nuts and rice cakes every two hours to maintain energy through the day. For the other two meals of the day, eat whole grains (such as brown rice, pasta, millet, quinoa), potatoes, meat, fish, dried beans, vegetables, salads and occasionally low fat cheeses. Nobody 'needs' a dessert. Forget they exist except for special occasions. Avoid fruit straight after a meal if you suffer from intestinal wind and bloating.

Coping with mid-morning and afternoon energy slumps

It is the mid-morning and mid-afternoon slumps in energy that send people off to the coffee machine or reaching for a chocolate bar, when what they really need is a break from sitting, a relief from boredom or a short nap. Ironically, fatigue is made worse by the consumption of sugar, caffeine and chocolate as they all have this swing high, swing low effect on blood sugar. I have known many people who discover that they don't feel so tired if they exclude these substances from their diet and that afternoon fatigue is made even worse if they drink coffee, tea or eat sugary foods in the morning. If you really can't give up your daily cuppa, save it for the middle of the afternoon when you might really need it.

Karen's story

"I work long hours. I eat lunch about 12 o'clock, and then nothing again until I get home about 7.30 in the evening. I thought this was the way to lose weight, but then I found I was getting in from work and nibbling on cheese, biscuits, crisps and chocolate because I was starving hungry. This spoilt my appetite so my evening meal was a disaster, and then I would be going back to the fridge all evening, right until bedtime. I needed to lose about 3 kilos, but just couldn't shift them.

Since having an afternoon snack around 4 p.m. of crispbreads spread with almond spread, seeds, nuts and raisins with a cup of very weak green tea, I arrive home feeling just ready for my evening meal. I nibble on a raw carrot while I am preparing one of the meal suggestions in your Seven Day Meal Planner, and when I have eaten I feel satisfied. I go for a walk after dinner, whatever the weather and go to bed having digested my food properly. I sleep better and wake up refreshed, and just as important, lost 3 kg without even trying."

Fibre

Eating foods that contain fibre gives a feeling of fullness which combats the hunger of low blood sugar. Some foods contain a form of fibre called soluble fibre that enters the blood stream and helps keep blood sugar levels elevated. In particular, oats and pulses contain soluble fibre and can be added to the diet in the form of porridge oats, oat cakes and biscuits, beans in salads and stews, and as vege-bean burgers and dips. Apples contain pectin which is a form of soluble fibre so is also good for blood sugar.

Don't forget protein and complex carbohydrates

Make sure you have some kind of protein with each meal and at each snack. Protein foods are meat, fish, eggs, nuts, seeds, pulses (beans), tofu, cheese and yoghurt. Complex carbohydrates are found in whole grains (brown rice, brown pasta, oatmeal porridge and wholemeal bread), fruits, vegetables, seeds, nuts and pulses. The Seven Day Meal Planner will give you a good idea of how to balance your meals for even blood sugar control.

A lot of women have told me that when they have tried diets that recommend eating only fruit in the morning and nothing else until lunchtime they feel terrible, light headed, sick and unable to concentrate. The reasoning behind eating only fruit before midday is that the body is detoxifying in the morning, and fruit aids the detoxification process. Women who are suffering from disglycaemia usually can't handle only fruit in the morning until they have got their blood sugar back under control. I find that fruit combined with seeds and nuts gets round the lack of 'substance' to a fruit breakfast, still feels light and cleansing, and keeps blood sugar levels normal.

Withdrawal fatigue

Ironically, the first thing people notice when they change their eating habits and cut out nutritional stressors is that initially they feel very tired. This is because the adrenals are so used to being kick-started into action that it takes time to readjust to functioning normally. Give in to the fatigue, cancel all social engagements, go to bed earlier and get more sleep to get through this readjustment period. It can take between one and two weeks to feel the body's natural energy re-emerge.

149

Supplements

Even if you eat an excellent diet that contains no sugar or stimulants, you can help speed up your recovery by supplementing with a good B complex, vitamin C, and the minerals chromium, magnesium, zinc, calcium and manganese. All these nutrients are important in helping regulate blood sugar control and in creating energy from food. Chromium is especially important for eliminating cravings. I recommend 400 mcg per day of chromium polynicotinate for the first month with a maintenance of 200 mcg per day thereafter for women with cravings and poor blood sugar control.

L-glutamine, an amino acid, provides fuel directly to the brain, so helping eliminate the low blood sugar sensation. It can be taken as a supplement.

CHAPTER 14
DIGESTION, ABSORPTION & ELIMINATION

There is more to health than just eating the right food. You are not what you eat, but what you can digest, absorb and eliminate. As all good health starts in the digestive tract, that is the first place to start if you want to regain your health and vitality.

Stomach acid

When you eat food the digestive process starts in the mouth with the release of amylases from the salivary glands to start the breakdown of carbohydrates. Food reaching the stomach enters a highly acidic environment. Stomach acid is there to kill off bacteria in food and to break down proteins into smaller particles. It also stimulates peristaltic action, that is the muscular contractions of the intestines that push waste matter along ready for elimination. At the same time, minerals attached to the proteins are released ready for absorption in the intestine.

Reduction in stomach acid is common in women who are under stress and eating a poor diet, especially one deficient in zinc and vitamin B6, both of which are needed to produce stomach acid. Symptoms of low stomach acid include a feeling of heaviness in the stomach after eating, bloating, belching and ironically, acidity in the stomach. When acid levels fall too low, the stomach sometimes over compensates by producing too much acid, leading to acid reflux and burning sensation in the stomach (heartburn).

If you are not sure if you are suffering from low acid stomach, next time you get indigestion or heartburn, trying swallowing the juice of half a lemon diluted in a glass of luke warm water. If it brings instant relief, then you can take a supplement of weak stomach acid called betaine hydrochloride for a few months. You will know if you need the supplement or not because you will experience a warm sensation in the stomach if you don't need it, and no sensation at all if you do (chapter 10).

Because low stomach acid leads to a depletion of minerals, women can suffer from iron, calcium and zinc deficiency. Many symptoms associated with hormone disharmony are usually due in part to zinc deficiency. With normal absorption of minerals women notice that very quickly their nails get stronger, their hair stops falling out, their skin takes on a healthy glow and they feel calmer and more energetic.

Digestive enzymes

After leaving the stomach, the soup-like contents, called chyme, enter the upper intestine and are worked upon by pancreatic enzymes and bile. Their role is to break down carbohydrates and fats, and reduce the protein chains into even smaller particles. Fats, carbohydrates, proteins, vitamins and minerals are absorbed through the intestinal wall. Waste matter, including cholesterol and hormones, is excreted via the colon.

Women with hormone problems very often have digestive problems too. Adding digestive enzymes, as well as betaine hydrochloride, to their supplement programme makes sure that all food is properly digested.

Fibre, detoxification and hormones

Fibre is important for excreting excess hormones from the body. When hormones are produced, they do a circuit around the body once, fulfilling their role in the process. They then travel to the colon for excretion. If there is not enough fibre in the colon, there is a risk of the waste matter stagnating and used hormones, particularly oestradiol, being reabsorbed into the blood and reactivated. This can play havoc with hormone levels and sensitivity to your own hormones.

In his book, "*The Optimum Nutrition Bible*", Patrick Holford tells us that rural African dwellers eat about 55 grams of dietary fibre a day, compared with the UK average of 22 grams. They also have the lowest incidence of bowel diseases. An ideal intake is 35 grams or more. Fibre is essential for the health of the colon (the body's waste disposal unit). It keeps faecal matter moving and avoids stagnation. A stagnating colon is like a dirty sewer. Stagnation leads to bowel problems such as colitis, diverticulitis, appendicitis and bowel cancer. The Seven Day Meal Planner shows you how to incorporate fibre naturally into your diet with delicious, unrefined, wholesome foods.

Constipation

Most people in the west are constipated, even if they 'go' once a day. The definition of constipation is a 'transit time' (the length of time it takes for the food you eat to travel the full length of your gastrointestinal tract) of more than 24 hours. The colon is designed to remove waste matter within between 12 and 24 hours after food has been eaten. If you want to check your transit time, swallow whole or only partially chew a teaspoon of sweet corn and watch to see when it appears the other end!

With insufficient fibre over the years the inside of the colon becomes caked with compacted faecal matter, reducing the diameter of the colon and reducing the amount of nutrients that can be absorbed.

As well as insufficient fibre, some foods can actually encourage a clogging up of the colon. Dairy produce and meat can be quite mucous forming and can cause an upset in bowel function. This is particularly so for people with a dairy produce sensitivity. Wheat can also have a similar effect due to its rather sticky protein, gluten, which is especially high in European bread where extra gluten is added for better rising. Personally, I find that chocolate, especially the pure, dark plain chocolate, is good at clogging up the colon and is therefore best avoided.

Stagnation and autotoxicity

A 'clogged up' colon does not just lead to bowel disease. We all carry around a bacteria population in the gut, some good, some bad. The late Dr. Barnard Jensen, chiropractor and pioneer for over 60 years in the field of natural health,[139] tells us that stagnating faecal matter encourages a population of bacteria who happily feed on it, producing toxins as a by-product of their metabolism. The toxins are absorbed through the colon membrane into the bloodstream and travel around the body, turning it into a *"dump for toxic waste"*. This puts a strain on the liver (the organ of detoxification), the adrenals and the immune system, resulting in poor, spotty skin, bad breath, lethargy, headaches, hormonal imbalance and more infections.[140] The best dietary sources of fibre are fruits, vegetables, nuts, seeds, pulses and wholegrains, particularly oats.

Intestinal flora

Having the right balance of gut bacteria (intestinal flora) is important for processing hormones to ensure that they are not reactivated or reabsorbed. Most women with hormonal problems have low levels of good intestinal flora, which in turn can lead to a proliferation of yeasts and fungi. Friendly bacteria produce antibiotics, B vitamins and vitamin K. They also deactivate cholesterol and hormones.

Colon cleanse

A periodic colon cleanse can keep the colon clean and working efficiently. A colon cleanse involves taking psyllium husks, often combined with, guar gum, pectin and specialised herbs. Colon cleansing products are available and should be used along side an alkaline, non-mucous forming, detoxifying diet for about two to four weeks.

A colon cleanse is quite different to colonic irrigation which involves introducing warm water at high pressure into the colon to "pressure clean" the colonic debris. While this can be a very quick and efficient way of cleaning the colon, it is invasive and many women prefer to take a more gentle and non-invasive route to colonic health.

Help for a sluggish colon

If you exercise regularly and eat a wholefood diet, avoiding the foods that clog the colon and you still have a sluggish colon, the following supplements can help persuade your colon into good elimination habits.

- Acidophilus (friendly gut bacteria) can be obtained from live yoghurt in small quantities, or you can take a supplement. Look for supplements that do not contain *lactose* if you are milk intolerant.

- Psyllium husks, taken as capsules or powder, are a neutral form of fibre that help bulk out the contents of the colon and speed up elimination of waste matter.

- Magnesium as citrate or gluconate (100 – 300 mg per day) helps to relax the muscles of the colon if they have 'seized up'. If you get muscle spasms or cramping, often associated with irritable bowel syndrome, magnesium can bring almost instant relief (often within twenty minutes).

- Vitamin C taken to 'bowel tolerance', i.e. when bowel movements become loose, is an effective way to kick start a stubborn colon into action. Take in powder form as magnesium ascorbate (buffered ascorbic acid to avoid acidity in the digestive tract). Some of my clients have needed to start with six scoops of magnesium ascorbate, i.e. six grams, to get things moving. However, over time, as the colon becomes accustomed to new dietary habits, increased levels of exercise and fibre, my clients have been able to reduce that amount to a 1,000 mg (1 gram) tablet of vitamin C per day, and still maintain colon function.

- Exercise is essential for keeping calcium in the bones. It is also vital for keeping the colon moving. A 30 – 40 minute brisk walk every day, jumping/running on the spot, skipping or dancing have all been shown to be effective at reducing stress, relieving constipation as well as protecting against heart disease and osteoporosis.

CHAPTER 15
NUTRITIONAL DEFICIENCES AND
DIETARY SUPPLEMENTS

Nutritional deficiencies

Women suffering from hormonal distress invariably have some nutritional deficiencies. Eating a wholefood diet with only the occasional nutritional stressors will go a long way to ensuring that you are getting the right level of nutrients, especially if you eat organic wherever possible. Lack of certain nutrients are linked to particular symptoms associated with hormone distress.

The following is a guide to the predominating nutritional deficiency with regard to symptoms. Please do not make the mistake of taking one nutrient in large quantities. In nutrition the whole is greater than the parts. In other words, all the nutrients provided by nature in the food you eat work together. There is a real danger of supplementing with say vitamin B6 or calcium or iron on their own, without the other nutrients that help to make them effective in the job they do. You can cause even greater deficiencies in the other nutrients by taking just one nutrient out of context.

B vitamins

B vitamins are important in the creation of energy, in helping the liver to convert harmful oestrogens to oestriol ready for excretion in the colon, in improving immunity, and in balancing moods. They are particularly helpful if you are suffering from depression, anxiety or irritability. The predominant B vitamin deficiencies in hormonal distress are vitamins B3 and B6. Water retention is a classic symptom of B6 deficiency, as is tingling in the hands and fingers.

Magnesium and vitamin D

Lack of magnesium and vitamin D can lead to calcium imbalance. Symptoms associated with lack of magnesium are muscle cramping (period pains as well as leg cramps), irritability, insomnia and high blood pressure.

Chromium and manganese

Both chromium and manganese are vital for balancing blood sugar levels. These nutrients are especially important for someone suffering from fluctuations in blood sugar control or disglycaemia. Chromium helps to control cravings for sweet things and other nutritional stressors. If you suffer from blood sugar problems and joint pain, particularly problems with cartilage, you may well need some more manganese as manganese is also required for cartilage production.

Zinc

Zinc is required by the enzymes that manufacture hormones. It works hand in hand with vitamin B6 which cannot do it's job properly without zinc. Check your nails, if you have white spots on your nails, then you are certainly suffering from zinc deficiency. PMS, menopausal symptoms, poor skin condition (especially acne), poor immunity and fatigue are also signs of zinc deficiency.

Vitamins A, C and E.

These are all required in the manufacture of hormones and are important anti-oxidants to protect essential fatty acids. Vitamins C, E and hesperidin (part of the vitamin C complex) can be very helpful in treating breast tenderness and for hot flushes. Vitamin C requirement soars with a rise in stress levels.

Boron

Boron is a mineral needed by the body to stimulate the production of small amounts of oestrogen from the adrenal glands after the ovaries have stopped production. It also reduces the rate of calcium excretion in the urine. A lack of boron has been associated with osteoporosis.

Iodine and iron

Iodine is important for thyroid health, which is intrinsically linked to hormone health. The thyroid check list in chapter 8 will give you an idea of whether or not you are suffering from low thyroid function.

Women are notoriously short of iron, especially if they have heavy periods. Pale skin, fatigue, breathlessness on exertion, loss of appetite, nausea and sore tongue are all symptoms of iron deficiency – even when blood tests appear to be normal (individuals can have different requirements outside the average normal range).

Selenium

Selenium is required in antioxidising enzymes that protect against cancer. Selenium is antagonistic to mercury. If you have amalgam fillings containing mercury, or you eat ocean caught fish regularly, you may need to think about taking a supplement containing selenium. I have also found selenium with vitamin E to be effective in cases of acne. Daily requirement for selenium is between 100 mcg and 200 mcg.

"But you can get everything you need from a well balanced diet!"

Diet, exercise and general lifestyle play an important part in creating hormonal harmony, whatever your age. However, there are times when supplementation of all the important vitamins, minerals, essential fatty acids and the use of herbal preparations can make an enormous difference to how you feel. The role of nutritional supplements is to supplement a good diet to make up a deficit that has probably been growing over many years. Specific herbal and phytohormone preparations can help correct imbalances in the endocrine system and block the ability of exogenous (produced outside the body) oestrogens from causing havoc with your hormone balance.

People observe, quite rightly, that taking pills and tablets is totally unnatural. But it isn't natural to eat, drink and breathe chemicals, or sit all day long surrounded by electromagnetic fields, in artificial lighting and air conditioning, not getting enough sleep, rest or exercise. I use supplements in my practice to counterbalance all the unnatural stressors to which women are exposed daily and to rebalance the deficit in nutrients that have built up over time.

Speeding up the healing process

As a society, we have all been brought up on quick fixes. Naturally people want to see quick results when they start a nutrition programme. They want to start feeling better within days, at the most a week or two. If they don't start feeling better, they lose faith in their body's natural ability to heal itself. Combining dietary manipulation with supplementation brings about a speedy relief from symptoms and encourages people to stick to their programme. I liken it to topping up each bucket of nutrients so that when they are full the body is able to take all the nutrients it needs without skimping and having to make do. This makes the healing process far more efficient.

If dietary supplements didn't work, I wouldn't recommend them. Good quality supplements are expensive and it can be a real pain having to remember to take several capsules or tablets every day. However, the results are usually worth the hassle and expense. I would like to see nutritional medicine made available on prescription.

Below are the supplements I have found to be the most effective in getting hormones back in balance.

Vitamins and minerals

I normally recommend a good quality 'core' multi vitamin and mineral supplement and 'add on' individual nutrients as necessary, according to the severity of the symptoms being experienced. Optimum quantities of nutrients for achieving hormonal health are listed below.

Vitamin A (as retinol and beta carotene)	2,500 – 7,500 i.u.s
B complex	25 – 100 mg
Folic acid	400 mcg
Vitamin B12	25 – 100 mcg
Vitamin C + bioflavinoids	500 mg–2,000 mg
Vitamin D	400 – 800 i.u.s
Vitamin E	400 – 800 i.u.s
Boron	1.5 – 3 mg
Calcium citrate	100 mg - 600 mg
Chromium polynicotinate or as GTF	100 - 200 mcg
Iron citrate	14 – 18 mg
Iodine	50 – 150 mcg
Magnesium citrate	100 mg - 600 mg
Manganese	5 - 20 mg
Selenium	100 – 200 mcg
Zinc citrate	15 – 20 mg

Table 4. Optimum levels of nutrients for hormone related health problems

Macro minerals, like calcium and magnesium, have to be taken separately as sufficient amounts cannot be contained in a multi vitamin and mineral complexed supplement. If you have very heavy periods or have been shown to have an iron deficiency, then you may need to take extra iron.

Vitamins C and E can be taken separately for therapeutic treatment of hot flushes and breast tenderness up to the maximum quantities shown in table 4. Vitamins A and D can be taken as extra in fish liver oil during winter months or if you do not have daily access to sunshine during the spring and summer. An extra B complex can be taken to meet the quantities recommended if you are feeling very stressed, depressed, anxious, nervous or jittery.

158

Not all supplements are the same

"I take a multi vitamin and mineral supplement bought from a pharmacy. I can't say I feel any better for it and I think I have wasted my money." Bridget T, Interpreter

Many popular over the counter supplements really aren't worth the money spent on them. They contain inadequate amounts of nutrients in forms that the body cannot use. These supplements also contain additives, sugar, yeast, colourings and inorganic forms of minerals, usually sulphates, oxides and carbonates in larger quantities than the body is used to dealing with. Better forms of minerals are gluconates, citrates, ascorbates, malates and amino acid chelated.

You can actually save yourself a lot of disappointment - and money - by investing in a visit to a qualified practitioner trained in nutrition. You will be recommended appropriate supplements as part of a comprehensive nutrition programme (please see page 189 to find out more about *'distance consultations'* via email, phone and post).

A good supplement programme is designed to meet the following criteria:

- It matches your specific need for nutrients
- All the nutrients are there for a particular purpose
- They interact with each other for increased efficacy
- They will not upset you even if you are very sensitive
- They do not contain any additives that will aggravate your health problems
- Herbs and important nutrients work together to encourage the body's own healing ability

It is important that you talk to your doctor before taking any kind of supplements if you are already taking prescribed medication. A good nutritional therapist will be able to advise you about supplements if you are pregnant or planning to become pregnant.

Essential fatty acids

The role of essential fatty acids (EFAs) is explained in more detail in chapter 12. Supplements of GLA are obtained from evening primrose oil, borage (starflower) oil, and blackcurrant oil. The omega-3 fatty acids, including EPA and DHA are usually obtained from linseed oil and fish oil. Linseed oil contains predominantly omega-3 fatty acids which must then be converted to EPA and DHA in the body. Fish oil contains omega-3 fatty acids as well as EPA and DHA readily available for use by the body.

Be careful about buying oils containing EFAs. These oils are highly unstable and have to be properly prepared to ensure they stay fresh even after packaging. I have had bad reactions, including spotty skin and stomach ache, from taking evening primrose oil and fish oil that were not perfectly fresh. Essential fatty acids should not be exposed to light, heat or oxygen. Some companies use special containers instead of glass to reduce the possibility of damage. Free radicals are created when oils start to deteriorate, so only buy the very best quality organic EFAs and keep all oil-based supplements in the fridge.

Don't cook with linseed oil

A number of my clients have bought linseed oil that recommends them to use it in salad dressings and for cooking. Please do not use linseed oil for cooking! It is highly unstable and will create free radicals when heated. It will also lose much of its benefit in terms of essential fatty acids.

Natural plant hormone regulators

In chapter 2, I talked about the power of plant oestrogens, or phytoestrogens. These are found in a wide variety of foods including soya, citrus fruits, wheat, liquorice, alfalfa, celery, seaweed and fennel.

Other plants that contain phytohormones

Red clover, hops, celery seed, alfalfa, liquorice root, rhubarb, fennel and ginseng - all can help to alleviate period pains, regulate periods, reduce spotting, hot flushes, night sweats and vaginal dryness. Many are available in women's supplements to help with the symptoms of menopause.

Natural progesterone

Natural progesterone is obtainable on prescription as a cream in the U.K. and orally or as a gel in Belgium. Dr. John Lee brought natural progesterone to public awareness after using it successfully on his menopausal patients and those with osteoporosis (chapter 9). It is also useful for treating women who have had breast cancer to stop recurrence of the disease as it helps to address the oestrogen dominance that may have led to the cancer developing in the first place. And it can be helpful in treating fibroids, cysts and endometriosis.

Indole-3-Carbinol (13C)

This is a phytochemical isolated from cruciferous vegetables (i.e. broccoli, cauliflower, brussels sprouts, turnips, kale, green cabbage, mustard seed) that is showing promise as an anti-cancer agent. If you want to help prevent breast and cervical cancer, you really do need to eat up your greens![141,142,143]

Isoflavones

Isoflavones are phytoestrogens that are particularly high in fermented soya products. Some studies show that isoflavones help with symptoms of menopause, increase bone density and protect against heart disease and breast cancer.[144,145,146,147] You can take isoflavones from fermented soya as a supplement in either pill, tablet or powder form. This is especially useful if you hate the taste of tofu or are soya sensitive.

Herbs to restore hormone balance

According to Thorsons *"Guide to Medical Herbalism"*, the following herbs have been used widely through the ages for female problems.[148]

Vitex agnus castus (chaste berry)

Vitex agnus castus has a normalising and regulatory effect on the pituitary gland. It regulates periods, helps with heavy bleeding, too-frequent or painful periods, alleviates PMS, reduces hot flushes, and can increase the ratio of progesterone to oestrogen by balancing excess oestrogen.

Black cohosh, dong quai and wild yam

They have progesterone-favourable effects on the body. Wild yam is especially rich in diosgenin, from which progesterone can be made in the laboratory. While these plants may help to balance hormones, the body cannot turn these phytonutrients into progesterone itself. They therefore do not replace the need for progesterone in a person who is progesterone deficient. However, like the herbs, wild yam is a natural hormone balancer. It can raise oestrogen levels when they are low, and lower them when they are too high. It is also an antispasmodic and is useful for painful periods.

All of these herbs can be very powerful in their action. Agnus castus is particularly good for helping restore absent periods, while phytoestrogens from red clover, hops, celery seed, alfalfa, liquorice root, rhubarb, fennel and ginseng are very effective for menopausal symptoms.

However, if your hormones are already pretty well balanced for your age and stage in life, then taking these hormone altering herbs can bring on the symptoms you were hoping to avoid. I found this out when I realised I was in perimenopuase and wanted to experiment with 'alternative HRT' (I don't recommend anything until I have tried it myself first). I didn't have any symptoms at that time apart from a drop in energy levels and some generalised food allergy symptoms. I started using wild yam cream that contained red clover, black cohosh, dong quai and vitex agnus castus. Within a week I was experiencing hot flushes and night sweats. I stopped using the cream immediately!

A year later, during the summer when I was feeling rather hot all the time at night and my sleep was being disturbed, I tried taking isoflavones. This time I felt extremely irritable and found myself snapping at my nearest and dearest. Proof indeed that these natural substances are powerful enough to raise oestrogen levels. In the end, I discovered natural progesterone cream to be the answer for me over a period of about a year when my hormones were fluctuating the most. When I used natural progesterone cream, I felt stable and calm, had plenty of energy and slept well at night (except in very hot weather). The trick is to experiment and discover what suits you best. It may be different from one person to the next, and can vary at different stages of your menopause.

Aiding detoxification - Silymarin (milk thistle)

Milk thistle is a 'hepatic' herb, i.e. it helps the liver to stay healthy. Milk thistle promotes regeneration of diseased liver cells and protects them against some poisons. It will also help with gall bladder problems. If you are taking HRT, the Pill or any other kind of medication for your hormone problems, using milk thistle will make sure that your liver carries out its important job of detoxification more efficiently and it will be protected from possible side effects from the medication itself.

CHAPTER 16
PUTTING IT ALL INTO PRACTICE

Putting into practice all your nutritional good intentions can initially be difficult for a lot of people. Most women don't have time or energy to plan, shop and prepare meals for themselves. They eat out a lot or they rely on canteen lunches and prepared meals from the supermarket. When they do cook, most people go for meals based around pasta, bread and cheese – convenience foods that are quick and easy to prepare.

For women living alone, healthy eating seems to present even more of a challenge. They tell me that when they are only cooking for one, it's not worth all the trouble. My response is, "You are worth the trouble!" Do start thinking of yourself as the most important person in your life. If you don't bother to take care of yourself, no-one else is going to do it for you.

Get organised

The truth is that there is no easy way round food and food preparation. They have to be prioritised back into people's lives. Human beings have some very fundamental needs for survival: fresh air, clean water, shelter, healthy food, adequate sleep, rest and exercise, rewarding activity and nurturing relationships. In today's fast paced life, women are being forced to choose work and financial reward over a healthy, balanced lifestyle. If you are to regain and maintain good health, you have to rebalance your life to make food one of the main priorities. The secret here is to get organised. Here are a few tips to help you on your way.

Make a shopping list

Make a shopping list before you go shopping. Have a running list in your kitchen. As you run out of things, jot them down so you don't forget. Use the shopping list provided as a starter.

Schedule two shopping trips per week

Aim to do one big shop per week, say at the weekend if that is when you have the most time, and one shop during the week, either at lunchtime or on your way home from work. Don't go home first, or you won't feel like going out again, especially not to shop. Get into a routine so that you don't have to think too much about shopping. It becomes part of your weekly schedule, just as going to work or going out for a meal might do.

Prepare food in batches

When you prepare food make big batches so you don't have to cook from scratch every day. Have something prepared in advance for the days when you have to work late, go to the gym or visit friends. For example, make a big salad, saucepan of soup, large batch of potatoes or rice, a big bowel of ratatouille, curry or stews. Make enough for about three days. Once cooked, most things keep for a good three days covered and in the fridge, or you can freeze them. That way hunger won't take you by surprise and you find yourself snacking on unsuitable things.

Only buy healthy food

Only buy healthy foods that you know you will eat. If your failing is snacking on cheese, chocolate or biscuits when you get home from work, then don't have them in the house. Instead make a large hummus or aubergine dip and have some organic carrots ready scrubbed and eat those while you are preparing your evening meal.

Visualisation

Envisage at the start of each day what you want to eat. Plan your breakfast the day before, and make your lunch for the next day the evening before if you know you can't get healthy food at work. Use visualisation before going out in the evening. If you are going for a meal, picture yourself drinking either no wine, or just one glass if it's mid-week. Picture yourself saying 'no' to dessert, and 'yes' to salads, vegetables, jacket or boiled potatoes, and grilled or roasted meat and fish (depending on your tastes).

Using the Seven Day Meal Planner

Use the Seven Day Meal Planner and Recipes to get you started. It is not a diet to be followed religiously, but more of a guide to show you how to incorporate more fruit, vegetables, good quality protein and complex carbohydrates painlessly into your daily eating habits. There are no nutritional stressors in this eating plan.

The meals cater for vegetarians, meat and fish eaters, are very low in dairy produce and fairly low in wheat based foods. For example, I haven't included pasta, although if you have no intolerance to wheat you can substitute wholemeal pasta for potatoes when you feel like it. Sugar and processed fats are not included in this meal planner either. The emphasis is on naturally sweetened foods (for those who have a sweet tooth), on wholefoods and cold pressed oils.

Vegetarian and vegan alternatives

I have included vegetarian or vegan alternatives within all the daily suggestions and leave the choice to each individual's taste and lifestyle preference. In the end, the majority of people tend to go for a mixture - some days preferring predominantly vegetarian meals, other days needing to eat a piece of meat or fish. Go with what your body seems to be telling you – as you become rebalanced, you really will know what you need.

Basically this meal planner helps you to cut out all the potentially harmful foods that may be ruining your health. It acts as a guide to healthier eating habits until it becomes second nature to make appropriate choices. And most important, none of the meals takes long to prepare.

Ground seed and nut mix

For extra creamy goodness, adding ground seeds, with or without nuts, gives fruit shakes and breakfast cereals extra vitamins, minerals, protein and essential fatty acids. Refined breakfast cereals have all their goodness removed, and are then 'fortified' with one or two vitamins and minerals that don't replace anything like the number and quality of those removed. This ground seed and nut mixture is a form of natural food fortification. You can grind up three or four days worth and keep in an air tight jar in the fridge if you are short of time.

Use any combination of linseeds, sunflower seeds, pumpkin seeds, sesame seeds, almonds and cashew nuts.

What to spread on bread and toast

Olive oil on toast and bread is delicious. It can bring back memories of Mediterranean holidays, especially if you rub your bread with a clove of garlic, add some basil and some sun dried tomatoes. Or you could use organic butter if you have no dairy sensitivity.

The best alternatives to butter that work equally well on rice cakes, for those who are avoiding wheat and bread, are spreads made from seeds and nuts. Available from all good health food shops, they are in jars, look like peanut butter, but are made from different kinds of seeds and nuts, ranging from sesame seeds (tahini), sunflower seed, hazelnut, almonds, cashew nut, and all kinds of combinations of any of those. Choose the brands where the natural oils haven't been emulsified into the spread. You will see them easily – the oil sits on the top of the spread and you just stir it in. Old fashioned peanut butter was always like this until the manufacturers learnt to emulsify the oils and add sugar (or dextrose) and salt to what was once an excellent food. Keep all seed and nut butters in the fridge.

Baking

The best fats to use from a health point of view, are butter and olive oil. Some products now available from health food stores and major supermarket chains are based solely on naturally saturated plant oils, such as coconut and palm oil, that have not been hydrogenated. They are made from organically grown plants, contain no dairy produce and no chemicals or artificial colouring. As someone who doesn't make cakes, I can only advise experimenting with different kinds of fats for baking.

Do remember to use good quality unrefined flour for cakes, biscuits and desserts. To sweeten, you can use unheated honey in place of sugar. You can also use raw cane sugar, the really dark treacly kind that contains valuable minerals including iron. However, if you have a grain allergy, you may well be sensitive to cane sugar. If you have a wheat allergy, you will need to experiment with flours made from rice, quinoa, potato, corn, millet and buckwheat - or just give up the idea of eating bakery products altogether!

Sugar replacements

It's better to try and kick a sugar habit altogether. If you are trying to overcome cravings use dried fruits and almonds. Dried fruits are particularly nice on break-fast cereals or with fresh fruit salad and nuts in the morning, as well as being a good source of iron and calcium.

Do avoid artificial sweeteners. The most common one in use in most 'sugar-free' and diet products is aspartame. Aspartame is an excitotoxin that targets the central nervous system. The U.S. FDA has come up with a great long list of side effects from using aspartame that range from headaches through to Parkinson's disease, multiple sclerosis, seizures and death. The methanol in aspartame converts to formaldehyde when its temperature exceeds 30°C. Formaldehyde is classed with cyanide and arsenic, toxic to human beings. Do check labels carefully and don't give aspartame sweetened foods and drinks to children.[149,150]

Milk substitutes

There are a number of plant based alternatives to dairy milk. You can make your own nut milk, or take a look the different kinds of rice, oat and nut milk available in supermarkets and health food shops.

Nut milk

Try grinding up nuts, particularly cashews and almonds, in a coffee grinder to a fine powder and mixing with bottled water, or apple, grape or pineapple juice, to make a creamy 'nut milk' to drink on its own or to pour over fruit and puffed rice or maize. You can also buy nut milks in health food stores.

Coconut milk

As coconut contains caprylic acid which has anti-fungal properties, you could try soaking desiccated coconut in fruit juice or water and using the strained liquid as a milk substitute. The solids can be added to the seed and nut breakfast. Creamed coconut can also be used in this way. Or you can buy cans of prepared coconut milk for use in oriental cooking. Just dilute with bottled water and pour on cereals.

Rice and oat milk

Available from health food shops and a tasty substitute for cow's milk. Avoid oat milk if you have a sensitivity to gluten, as oats contain a small amount of gluten.

A note about soya milk

A lot of people use soya milk instead of cow's milk. However, there has been a lot of controversy about the possible harmful effects of using soya the way we do in the west. In the east, it is used in small quantities and always fermented. Soya exerts quite a powerful oestrogenic effect on the body, which is thought to be beneficial, but unfermented and in large quantities may actually be harmful. I therefore do not recommend soya milk in large quantities, especially as it can also cause intolerance in some people.

CHAPTER 17
THE SEVEN DAY MEAL PLANNER,
SHOPPING LIST AND RECIPES

Breakfasts - Choose from:

• **Porridge** made with oats or quinoa flakes and water. Add chopped fruit of your choice, seeds, nuts and rice milk if desired. If preferred you can stir in ground seed and nut mixture for natural sweetness and to give a creamy texture to the porridge. If you like a sweeter taste, add raisins or other chopped dried fruit.

• **Muesli** soaked overnight in water or fruit juice. Add a combination of chopped fresh fruit, almonds, sunflower, sesame and pumpkin seeds, and sun dried fruits. Pour on milk substitute of choice.

• **Banana** or any fruit of choice and a handful of sunflower or pumpkin seeds and almonds, cashews or walnuts – for people in a hurry or with little appetite for breakfast.

• **Crispy, sugar-free and gluten-free cereals** made from corn, quinoa, millet, or rice flakes (available from health food shops), with fresh fruit of choice, and almond, rice or oat milk, or fruit juice.

• **Dried fruit compote** made from dried fruit soaked in water and a little apple juice overnight. Top with toasted sesame or sunflower seeds, or toasted, chopped almonds. Be sure to buy unsulphured, sun dried fruit.

• **Fruit, seed and nut breakfast** (see recipe).

• **Milk-free fruit shake.** Liquidise a banana or any soft fruit of choice with equal quantities of fruit juice and mineral water and ground seed and nut mix. Drink immediately.

• **Organic yoghurt or cottage cheese** with chopped banana or any fruit of choice and ground seed and nut mix.

• **Wholemeal bread or toast** spread with seed and nut spreads as above.

• **Rice cakes** spread with tahini (sesame paste) or other seed and nut butters of choice. Add raisins for sweetness if desired.

For big appetites

- **Poached, scrambled or boiled egg** with wholemeal toast or rice cakes, or omelette made just with eggs (no milk). A good protein breakfast based on the traditional English breakfast is a great way to start a busy day if you need a lot of food in the mornings. However, as it is rather acidic due to the high protein content and no vegetables, I do not suggest this as a regular every day breakfast. Also beware frying in fat. Grill or cook in a non-stick pan with no extra fat added.

- **Baked beans on toast.** Use tinned white haricot beans and stir into home made tomato sauce (see recipe).

- **Rice, potatoes, cold meat, fish ....** It's only cultural that we eat cereals for breakfast. Go with your appetite and how you feel. If you feel 'acidic' when you wake up, then go for fruit and seeds. If you have an enormous appetite and need sustaining through a long day, go for a protein based breakfast. Check out how you feel after the meal – sleepy, energised, indigestion, clean, constipated or free flowing – this is the best way to know what is best for you.

To drink

Choose from hot water with or without a slice of lemon juice (choose lemons untreated after picking), herbal teas (especially fresh mint tea in the summer), very weak green china tea, or fresh fruit juice. Rooibos (red leaf) tea from S. Africa is caffeine free and available from good supermarkets or health food shops. It tastes a bit like ordinary black tea (but not a lot!).

Snacks

Snacks between meals should consist of one piece of fruit, a handful of sunflower or pumpkin seeds, almonds, hazelnuts, cashews or walnuts, and sun-dried figs, apricots or raisins and sultanas. You could also eat a rice cake either plain, or spread with seed and nut spreads. Once your blood sugar is under control, you will find you need to snack between meals far less often.

Lunch and dinner

Lunch and Dinner are interchangeable, depending on timetable and lifestyle.

One of these meals should be based on a mixed raw salad, and the other should be based on lightly cooked vegetables, according to the guidelines given below.

Choose vegetables in season to reduce the risk of overuse of chemicals used for forced growing.

Make salad dressing with cold pressed oils (see recipe) and use regularly on salads and vegetables for essential fatty acids.

The meal planner includes a source of protein and complex carbohydrate at each meal as well as being high in fruit and vegetables. This ensures that the meals are very well balanced.

DAY ONE

Lunch
Salad consisting of grated carrots, lambs' leaves and alfalfa spouts + half a ripe avocado + half a tin of tuna in brine or a small pot of cottage cheese or small portion of hummus (see recipe). Use home-made salad dressing and a sprinkle of fisherman's salad.

Dinner
Homemade vegetable soup (see recipe).

DAY TWO

Lunch
Mixed green salad, alfalfa sprouts, the other half of yesterday's ripe avocado + prawns or tinned tuna or sardines or hummus or tofu slices. Use home-made salad dressing and a sprinkle of fisherman's salad. Eat with cold brown rice or wholemeal bread.

Dinner
Chicken or tofu with stir fried vegetables (see recipe).

DAY THREE

Lunch
Rice salad (see recipe). Eat hot or cold with a grated carrot and mixed green salad. Use home-made salad dressing and a sprinkle of fisherman's salad.

Dinner
Salmon steak and vegetables (see recipe).

DAY FOUR

Lunch
Aubergine dip (see recipe) and fresh mint, with yesterday's rice salad. Eat with watercress and cherry tomatoes. Use home-made salad dressing and a sprinkle of fisherman's salad.

Dinner
Lamb and/or red kidney bean ragout (see recipe).

DAY FIVE

Lunch
Tinned mackerel or tuna in brine, with a salad containing endive or lettuce, grated carrot, watercress and bean sprouts. Serve with wholemeal pitta bread or small, sliced baked potato (hot or cold). Use home-made salad dressing and a sprinkle of fisherman's salad.

Dinner
Vegetable curry (see recipe)

DAY SIX

Lunch
Wholemeal sandwich spread with hummus + tuna fish in brine (if desired), and alfalfa sprouts. Eat with a small, green side salad. Use home-made salad dressing and a sprinkle of fisherman's salad.

Dinner
Oven cooked ratatouille (see recipe) with chicken or tofu slices or vege-bean balls (see recipe).

DAY SEVEN

Lunch
Olive oil potato salad (see recipe). Eat with a borlotti bean salad consisting of lettuce, chopped celery and grated carrot. Use home-made salad dressing and a sprinkle of fisherman's salad.

Dinner

Oven cooked trout and almonds (see recipe).

Desserts

There are no desserts as such. Fresh fruit can be eaten 1 - 2 hours after a meal to avoid both stomach and intestinal gas. Pineapple can sometimes work after a meal because it contains bromelaine which can help digest protein. Keep desserts for occasional use only.

Shopping list

- Raw almonds, cashew nuts, walnuts, hazelnuts, brazil nuts, sunflower seeds, pumpkin seeds, sesame seeds, linseeds and pine kernels

- Tahini, almond, hazelnut and sunflower spreads

- Organic butter, spreads made from unhydrogenated palm, coconut and sunflower oils.

- Sun-dried, unsulphured figs, apricots, raisins, sultanas, prunes, dried apple and dried pears.

- Fresh fruit in season

- Rice cakes, wholemeal bread and wholemeal pitta bread

- Herbs: mint, parsley, rosemary, coriander, basil, and Wakama powdered seaweed

- Green china tea, rooibos tea, other teas of choice, bottled mineral water. Water filter

- Oats, quinoa flakes, muesli and other wholegrain, sugar-free cereals

- Rice, oat, almond and coconut milk

- Salad ingredients (seasonal): green salad, watercress, alfalfa and bean sprouts, endives, lambs' leaves, avocado, tomatoes, celery, crispy seaweed flakes

- Cold pressed sunflower oil, cold pressed virgin olive oil, sesame oil, organic balsamic vinegar

- Vegetables (seasonal): potatoes, onions, carrots, garlic, ginger, red, green and yellow peppers, courgettes, aubergines, broccoli, savoy cabbage, mushrooms, baby sweet corn, mange tout peas, fresh seaweed

- Brown rice, quinoa, millet and buckwheat

- Lamb, salmon, trout, chicken, tinned tuna, sardines, mackerel and tofu.

- Soy sauce, vegetable stock cubes, bouillon, black bean sauce, curry paste and coconut milk

- Chick peas, brown or green lentils, red kidney beans, borlotti beans, white haricot beans and tinned tomatoes

THE HEALTH & VITALITY RECIPES

How to use the recipes

If you are a confident cook, then please use these recipes as ideas and rough guidelines. Follow the spirit, using good quality ingredients, organic where possible, with the emphasis on vegetables, but feel free to change the recipes according to seasonal availability and personal taste.

If you are not so confident in the kitchen, then you can follow these recipes faithfully until you have got the hang of substituting one ingredient for another, depending on what you forgot to buy last time you shopped!

Do have fun with these recipe ideas. If there is anything you hate here, ignore it. Eating is meant to be a pleasure. You should never feel you have to eat a particular food just because it is 'good for you'.

The recipes are in the order in which they appear in the meal planner with a few extra meal ideas at the end. Most of the recipes are fine for both vegans and vegetarians, and confirmed meat eaters will enjoy them. If you hate fish, or are allergic to it, then use cubed or sliced tofu, beans or vegebean balls in place of fish where appropriate.

Steamed vegetables

You will see that in some places I have suggested serving with steamed vegetables such as cabbage, brussels sprouts, broccoli or green beans. Steaming is a very easy way to cook vegetables that retains all of their flavour and goodness. You can buy a 'petal' steamer in any hardware store or the kitchenware section of most supermarkets. This is a stainless steel steamer that fits inside any sized saucepan. You just fill the saucepan with water to just below the bottom of the steamer so that the vegetables don't touch the water, and cook them for between 5 and 10 minutes, depending on how crispy you like your vegetables.

Fruit, seed and nut breakfast

Choose a combination of any of the following:
50 gms sunflower seeds
50 gms pumpkin seeds
50 gms pine kernels
50 gms linseeds
50 gms sesame seeds
50 gms almonds
50 gms walnut or pecans
50 gms hazelnuts
50 gms cashews
30 gms brazel nuts
Chopped sun dried fruit of choice, including raisins
Chopped fresh fruit in season
Fresh fruit juice of choice (not made from concentrate)

Make up a large fruit salad, pour on fresh fruit juice to cover the fruit. Keep covered in the fridge with cling film. It will keep for up to three days.

Mix all the seeds, nuts and dried fruit in another large bowl and keep covered in the fridge. This will keep for two to three weeks – at least until you have eaten them all up!

Each morning put a helping of the fruit in a breakfast bowl and sprinkle with the seed, dried fruit and nut mix according to appetite.

All nuts should be whole and in their brown skins, i.e. no blanched almonds or hazelnuts. Avoid broken walnut pieces.

Make sure dried fruit is sun dried and without the addition of sulphur dioxide or glucose. If the apricots are orange, they contain sulphur dioxide.

Hummus (chick pea dip)

1 can cooked chick peas rinsed and drained
1 clove garlic chopped
Juice of 1/2 lemon
1 teaspoon tahini
Sea salt and black pepper
Olive oil
Chopped fresh parsley and mint
Wholemeal pitta bread

Place chick peas in a food processor with the garlic and enough olive oil to make a coarse puree. Add the lemon juice, tahini, salt and pepper and make into a thick puree. Place in the middle of a plate of salad. Drizzle with olive oil and sprinkle with chopped parsley and mint. Serve with hot pitta bread or wholemeal bread.

Vegetable soup (serves up to 6 people)

2 onions diced
Grated fresh ginger (piece as big as a golf ball)
4 sticks celery chopped into small pieces
4 large carrots chopped into small pieces
2 medium sized potatoes or sweet potatoes chopped into small pieces
1 vegetable stock cube without MSG (monosodium glutamate) – (optional)
1 teaspoon miso dissolved in hot water (optional)
Sprinkle of powdered norri flakes (optional)
Black or white pepper
Pinch of sea salt
Fresh coriander chopped
1 tablespoon (approximately) cold pressed, virgin olive oil
Cooked chicken, can sweet corn, can borlotti beans (all optional)

In a large saucepan, cook the onions and ginger in the olive oil until onions are transparent. Add the celery, then the carrots and potatoes. Continue cooking for around five minutes in the oil. Add a little more oil if it all starts sticking. Dissolve the vegetable stock cube into a cup of boiling water along with the miso (optional) and add to the vegetables. Add pepper, powdered norri flakes and sea salt. Top up with plenty of water to around 2 cm above the vegetables.

If you are using a pressure cooker, put on the lid and bring to steam. Turn heat down and set timer for 10 minutes. In a saucepan, put on the lid, bring to the boil, turn heat down and simmer until all the vegetables are cooked (around 20 minutes).

Using a soup blender, blend all the ingredients to a smooth texture. You can leave some solid pieces of vegetable if preferred. Add more water if a thinner soup is desired. Stir in the sweet corn and/or borlotti beans (optional), plus the coriander, and add diced cooked chicken if desired. Heat through thoroughly. Pour into soup bowls and eat as a meal on its own or with fresh, wholemeal bread.

Stir fried vegetables with chicken or tofu (serves 2-4)

1 large onion chopped
I packet baby sweet corn chopped into two or three pieces each
1 packet mange touts peas
1/2 broccoli head with florets finely chopped
1 packet bean sprouts
1 cup of cashew nuts
1 tablespoon olive oil and 1 teaspoon sesame oil
1 tablespoon soy sauce or 2 tablespoons black bean sauce
1 wine glass of dry white wine
Chopped cooked chicken or tofu

Rinse and chop all the ingredients. Place the two kinds of oil in a large non stick frying pan or in a wok and heat enough to cook the ingredients, but not to smoking point. Add the onions and cook until transparent. Then add the sweet corn pieces and broccoli florets and cook for two to three minutes with the onions. Stir in the soy sauce or black bean sauce and cook for a further two minutes. Finally add the rest of the ingredients and cook for another two to three minutes, making sure the vegetables are still crisp and colourful. Serve with wholegrain rice.

Salmon steak with vegetables (serves 2)

2 fresh salmon steaks
1 medium sized courgette chopped
1/2 each of red, green and yellow or orange pepper chopped
Powdered norri flakes
Juice of 1/2 lemon
1 clove garlic crushed
Black pepper and a pinch of sea salt
Fresh thyme
Fresh seaweed or 1/2 fresh broccoli head
2 medium potatoes scrubbed
Olive oil

Place the two potatoes in a hot oven (200 - 220°C) for 30 - 45 minutes, or until cooked. Place the salmon steaks in a large oven proof dish and surround with the chopped courgette and peppers, garlic, fresh thyme and sea salt. Pour on the lemon juice and enough water to cover 1 cm over the bottom of the dish. Sprinkle the powdered norri flakes over the fish to give a generous covering and season with ground black pepper. Place in the hot oven about 20 minutes after the potatoes have gone in.

Cook the fresh seaweed in a pan of boiling water for two to three minutes just before the rest of the food is cooked, or steam the broccoli florets for 3 - 4 minutes. Remove fish from the oven and serve with the potato and fresh seaweed or broccoli. Drizzle olive oil and a pinch of sea salt on the baked potato.

Rice salad (serves 2-4)

1 cup wholegrain rice
2 cups of water
1/2 vegetable stock cube (without MSG)
1 onion chopped
1 clove garlic crushed
1 red or green pepper chopped
Small punnet of mushrooms washed and sliced
1 dessertspoon pine kernels and 6 walnuts
Juice of 1/2 a lemon
Fresh mint and parsley
Olive oil, sea salt and ground black pepper

Cook the rice in the water with the stock cube until tender. Meanwhile, chop and cook the onion, garlic, pepper and mushrooms in a little olive oil for about 5 minutes. Remove from the heat and stir in the rice, lemon juice, chopped mint and parsley. Sprinkle with walnuts and pine kernels.

Eat with a mixed green salad or a grated carrot and celery salad.

Aubergine and tahini dip

1 medium aubergine
1 clove garlic chopped
Juice of 1/2 lemon
1 teaspoon tahini
Sea salt and black pepper
1 tablespoon of olive oil
Chopped fresh parsley and mint
Wholemeal pitta bread

Bake the whole aubergine in the oven for about 30 minutes until soft. Remove skin and stems. Chop roughly and place in food processor with garlic and make a coarse puree. Add the lemon juice, olive oil, tahini, salt and pepper and make into a thick puree. Place in the middle of a plate of salad. Drizzle with olive oil and sprinkle with chopped parsley and mint. Serve with salad and hot pitta bread (if desired).

Lamb and/or red kidney bean ragout (serves 2-4)

400 g lean lamb fillet cubed
1 can cooked red kidney beans
2 large onions chopped
2 medium carrots chopped
2 sticks celery chopped
4 medium sized potatoes scrubbed and chopped
1 tablespoon bouillon or 1 vegetable stock cube (both optional)
Black pepper and sea salt
Olive oil
Chopped rosemary and mint
2 glasses red wine
Diced white or green cabbage or broccoli, or green salad

Heat the olive oil in a large saucepan and cook the onions until golden. Add the cubed lamb and cook until brown. Add the bouillon and cook for a further three minutes. Add the carrots, celery and potatoes, rosemary and mint, the red wine and black pepper, and sufficient water to just cover the ingredients. Cook until the potatoes and carrots are soft (about 20 - 30 minutes). If you are using tinned, i.e. pre-cooked, kidney beans instead of, or as well as the lamb, add those ten minutes before the end of the cooking time. Serve with a green salad or lightly steamed, diced cabbage.

Cous cous made with quinoa (serves 2 – 4)

1 cup quinoa
1/2 vegetable stock cube without MSG
1 tablespoon olive oil
1 onion chopped
1 clove garlic crushed
1 small punnet of mushrooms washed and sliced
2 tablespoons pine kernels
Juice of 1 lemon
Chopped fresh mint and parsley
Black pepper and pinch of sea salt

Cook 1 cup of quinoa with 2 cups of water until the seeds have softened and and all the water has been used up (about 20-30 minutes). Meanwhile, cook the onion and garlic in the olive oil. Add mushrooms and pine kernels and cook for 2 – 3 minutes. Add black pepper and sea salt. Cook for a further 2 – 3 minutes. Remove from the heat and add the lemon juice, half the mint and half the parsley. Serve either hot or cold with remaining parsley and mint and a green salad.

Vegetable curry with or without chicken or brown lentils (serves 2 – 4)

2 large onions chopped
1 piece of freshly grated ginger (golf ball size)
1 medium aubergine chopped
1 medium courgette chopped
1 packet baby sweet corn cut in two to three pieces each
2 tablespoons of either mild or medium curry paste
1 can of coconut milk
Olive oil

Chopped fresh coriander
2 cups of wholegrain basmati rice
Chopped cooked chicken (optional)
1 can of brown lentils, rinsed and drained

Cook the onions and ginger in olive oil until golden. Add the aubergine and baby sweet corn pieces and cook for two to three minutes. Add the curry paste and courgette and cook for another two to three minutes before pouring in the can of coconut milk and half of the chopped coriander. Stir and simmer until the aubergine is soft. Serve with rice and the rest of the coriander. If you are using cooked chicken or tinned lentils, add when you pour in the coconut milk.

Oven baked ratatouille with tofu slices (serves 2 – 4)

1 large onion chopped
1 large courgette chopped
2 cloves garlic crushed
2 large tomatoes finely chopped
1 red and 1 green pepper
1 tablespoon pine nuts
1 bay leaf
Fresh chopped basil, thyme and parsley
Olive oil
Sea salt and black pepper
Juice of 1/2 lemon
Tofu cut into slices about 1/2 cm thick

Arrange all the vegetables in an oven proof dish and lay the tofu slices on the top. Season with the herbs, salt, pepper and lemon juice, and drizzle olive oil over the tofu. Cook for 20 – 30 minutes in a hot oven (200°C). Turn the ingredients a couple of times during the cooking process. If vegetables dry out, add water to the bottom of the dish. The ratatouille is cooked when the courgettes are soft but not soggy. Serve with a baked potato drizzled with olive oil or brown rice.

You can use any vegetables in season and bake them in the oven as above.

Olive oil potato salad (serves 1 - 2)

4 medium sized potatoes scrubbed but not peeled
1 clove of garlic crushed
1 dessertspoon pine kernels
Squeeze of lemon juice
2 dessertspoons cold pressed olive oil
Sprinkle of chopped parsley
Sea salt and ground black pepper

Cut the potatoes into bite sized chunks and place in boiling water until soft.
Drain and allow to cool. Add the rest of the ingredients and mix together. Serve
with a mixed salad.

Trout with almonds (serves 1 – 2)

2 fresh trout (pink salmon trout or rainbow trout)
Wakama powdered norri flakes
Sea salt and black pepper
Juice of 1/2 lemon
Olive oil
Whole, unblanched almonds (about a handful)
Broccoli or green beans
2 potatoes scrubbed and in their skins

Place potatoes in a hot oven (200°C) and cook for 1 hour. Or cook for 10 minutes
in a microwave oven at highest temperature. Fifteen minutes before the potatoes
are due to be ready, cook the trout in a non stick pan with a trace of olive oil,
powdered seaweed, black pepper, sea salt, lemon juice, and whole, unblanched
almonds. Cook both sides. Serve with steamed broccoli or green beans and a
jacket potato drizzled with olive oil.

You could also place the trout and almonds in the oven and cook for about twenty
minutes at 220°C.

Additional recipes

The following are some additional recipes to stretch the seven day meal planner for a few more days.

Potatoes with mustard sauce and borlotti beans (serves 2 – 4)
(This only works with firm potatoes such as Nicola, Cyprus new potatoes or Charlotte. It does not work with more floury English potatoes. You also need to use a firm bean like borlotti or kidney beans.)

4 medium potatoes cut in four
A bunch of spring onions sliced
1 – 2 tablespoons of wholegrain Dijon mustard
2 tablespoons olive oil
2 cloves garlic crushed or grated
1 can borlotti or kidney beans drained
Sea salt and ground black pepper
1 tablespoon sesame seeds
1 tablespoon sesame oil
Fresh coriander or parsley chopped

Boil or steam potatoes until just tender. Drain and put to one side. In a large frying pan or wok cook the onions for about 1 minute in the oil. Then add the garlic and cook for a few seconds longer. Add the potatoes, stirring well, then the beans, and finally the mustard and the sesame oil. Cook until everything is well heated through then sprinkle with sesame seeds and coriander or parsley. Serve with lightly steamed green vegetables or a green salad.

Quinoa (serves 2-3)

Quinoa can be cooked like rice and used in place of rice for a change. Cook one cup of quinoa to two cups of water. Bring to the boil and cook for 20 – 30 minutes over a low heat, until soft and fluffy. Serve in place of rice.

Home made meat balls (serves 2-3)

300 – 500 g lean minced lamb, pork or beef
2 medium onions finely chopped
1 dessertspoon tomato puree
1 teaspoon bouillon (liquid stock)
Fresh thyme, oregano or marjoram finely chopped
Sea salt and black pepper
Sesame seeds

Mix all the ingredients (except the sesame seeds) well together in a bowl with your hands. Shape them into meat balls and roll in the sesame seeds. Cook on a tray in a hot oven (180 – 200°C) for about 20 minutes. Serve with oven sauté potatoes, home made tomato sauce and a mixed salad.

Vege-bean balls

1 can of kidney beans and 1 can of brown lentils drained and rinsed
Wholemeal bread crumbs
Bunch spring onions washed and finely chopped
1 dessertspoon tomato puree
Fresh thyme, oregano or marjoram, mint and parsley finely chopped
Sea salt and black pepper
Olive oil
Sesame seeds

Put the beans in a blender and blend with the breadcrumbs into a paste. Place in a bowl with all the other ingredients (except the sesame seeds) and mix with your hands thoroughly. Shape into balls and roll in the sesame seeds. Cook in a hot oven (180 - 200°C) and serve with the home made tomato sauce, oven sautéd potatoes and lightly steamed vegetables or mixed salad.

Oven sauté potatoes

2 large potatoes scrubbed and cut into chunks (leave their skins on)
1 tablespoon olive oil
Sea salt and black pepper
Chopped fresh parsley and mint

Place all the ingredients in an oven proof dish and cook in a hot oven (200 - 250°C) for about 20 - 25 minutes.

Home made tomato sauce

1 medium finely chopped onion
1-2 cloves garlic crushed
Large can tomatoes
1 teaspoon bouillon (liquid stock) - (optional)
Fresh thyme, oregano or marjoram & 1 bay leaf
Tomato purée
Olive oil
Sea salt and black pepper
Cook the onions and garlic in olive oil until transparent. Add all the other ingredients and let them bubble gently until it is the required thickness (takes about 20 minutes).

Aubergine and chick peas (serves 2 – 4)

1 small can cooked chick peas drained and rinsed
1 small can tomatoes
1 small aubergine chopped
1 onion chopped
1 clove garlic grated or crushed
Juice of 1/2 lemon
Sea salt and black or white pepper
Olive oil
Fresh mint and parsley chopped

Cook the onion in a little olive oil in a saucepan or frying pan until transparent, about 3 – 5 minutes. Add the chopped aubergine and garlic and a little more olive oil. Cook for a further 5 minutes, or until aubergines are softened and browned. Add the chickpeas, tomatoes, lemon juice, half the mint and parsley, salt and pepper, and cook for a further 3 – 5 minutes, until thoroughly heated through. Sprinkle remaining mint and parsley over the mixture and serve with warm pitta bread or jacket potato and a seasonal salad.

Summer salad (makes a large bowl full)

1 small crisp lettuce and a few roquette leaves
Fresh basil
Red pepper finely chopped
2 carrots coarsely grated
Punnet of cherry tomatoes
2 celery sticks chopped
1/2 cucumber chopped
2 tablespoons sunflower seeds and 2 tablespoons sesame seeds

Mix all the ingredients in a large salad bowl and toss with the dressing below

----

Cold pressed oil salad dressing

Use three parts oil and one part vinegar. Of the oils use half sunflower and half olive oil. If you add linseed or other cold pressed oils for flavour, reduce the olive oil and sunflower oil to accommodate them. Do adapt this dressing to your own tastes.

Cold pressed sunflower oil
Cold pressed olive oil
A few drops of cold pressed hazelnut or walnut oil (optional)
1 tablespoon linseed oil
Balsamic or cider vinegar or juice of 1 lemon
Wholegrain mustard
Juice of 1 small orange (optional)
Pinch sea salt and black pepper
Chopped herbs of choice

Place all the ingredients in a screw top jar and shake well. You could put in a blender for a smoother finish. Keep in the fridge and use regularly on salads and vegetables for a good supply of essential fatty acids.

Other variations

You could add tofu and/or the ground seed and nut mix for a creamy salad dressing brimming with phytohormones.

For extra minerals and a taste of the sea, try adding Wakama powdered norri flakes or crispy seaweed flakes to your dressing. (Just experiment and use your dressing daily)

And garlic and cold pressed sesame oil tastes just great in a creamy salad dressing made with tofu.

CHAPTER 18
TAKE A (W)HOLISTIC VIEW OF HEALTH

Go with the flow. Worry only about the things you can change and not about the things outside your control. If life seems to be a struggle and a pile of stress, take some time to step back and reassess how you want to live your life for the least amount of stress and the most reward. It will no doubt mean making some changes in your life – job, relationships, diet, general lifestyle choices, like what time you go to bed, how you choose to exercise, priorities …

Getting your hormones back in balance through diet, lifestyle changes and supplementation can have a very positive effect on mood and energy. However, mind and body are so intrinsically linked that if you feel you are being pulled down and affected by unresolved stress, then it is worth investigating this with a qualified therapist.

Your hormones can even be influenced by something as fundamental as early programming around what it is to be a woman, self image, motherhood, menstruation and the menopause. The holistic approach to health means looking at the whole being, not just the separate parts. Your early programming can have a profound effect on your physical health. With optimum nutrition you can help redress the biochemical imbalances that have occurred through a less than ideal lifestyle. However, if there is a fundamental underlying chronic emotional stress problem, maintaining good health can become a constant battle.

As yet, psychological counselling is outside my field of expertise. However, I have included some books I have found useful in the recommended reading list. They can help with insights, but really skilful psychotherapy can remove emotional blocks much more effectively than trying to go it alone. Your inner woman is crying out for your help. Getting in touch with her and providing her with compassion, love and nurturing can really make a difference in bringing all the parts of your being into one complete whole for genuine, long lasting health.

DISTANCE CONSULTATIONS

Taking advice from a qualified nutritional therapist can be a helpful step in regaining or attaining hormone harmony. Personal Health Development offers detailed nutrition consultations to people, wherever they are in the world. These distance consultations can be carried out via email or over the 'phone.

How does a distance consultation work?

When you get in contact for a consultation, you will be sent a nutrition programme questionnaire to fill in and send back either by fax or email. Your completed questionnaire provides comprehensive medical history and a means to assess your biochemical imbalances and the impact of diet and lifestyle on your health and nutritional requirements.

Analysis of the questionnaire uses the Personal Health Development *Five Point Systems Imbalance Analysis Programme* which assesses:

Digestion and absorption: Low stomach acid, digestive enzymes, leaky gut, allergies and food intolerance, candidiasis and parasites, and absorption of nutrients.

Elimination: Stagnating colon, autotoxicity, detoxification, gut flora and liver function.

Blood sugar control: Energy and fatigue, stress, mental and emotional wellbeing, hormone disruption and cardiovascular health.

Endocrine Balance: Thyroid, pituitary and adrenal function, immune system, men's and women's hormone health.

Dietary and lifestyle habits: Alkalinity and acidity balance, nutritional stressors, nutritional deficiencies, balance of proteins, carbohydrates and fats, processed foods.

Other requirements for the consultation

You will need to provide a list of any supplements (herbs, vitamins, minerals, oils etc) that you are currently taking, including the brand name, type and quantity of nutrients or herbs in the supplement, for example, *"Blogs calcium carbonate 1200 mg"*. It's not enough to say that you are taking calcium or vitamin C, as all supplements are different in the quality and quantity of their contents.

Medical check up first

Before embarking on a nutrition programme you must have been for a check up with your own medical practitioner or specialist at least some time in the recent past.

What you get out of a consultation

What you will get out of the consultation is a comprehensive, tailor-made nutrition and supplement programme in the form of a spiral bound booklet that includes meal planners and recipes, food and symptoms diaries, background information and practical advice on how to apply the recommendations. This can be emailed or sent in the post, depending on your preference.

You will also receive free follow up via email for any questions you may have for one month following the consultation.

Getting in touch

If you would like more information about distance consultations, you can contact Carolyn Moody at phd@skynet.be, telephone 00 32 478 56 52 82 or via the Personal Health Development website at www.optimumnutrition.org.

RECOMMENDED READING

- *"Natural Hormone Health"*, Arabella Melville PhD, Thorsons, 1990

- *"Beat PMT through Diet"*, Maryon Stewart, Ebury Press, 1990

- *"Passage to Power"*, Leslie Kenton; Vermillion, 1996

- *"Natural Alternatives to HRT"*, Marilyn Glenville, Greenwich Editions, 1998

- *"The Breast Cancer Prevention & Recovery Diet"*, Suzannah Olivier, Michael Joseph, 1999

- *"Breast Health! The Wise Woman Way"*, Susun S. Weed, Ash Tree Publishing, 1996

- *"100% Health"*, Patrick Holford, Piatkus,1998

- *"The Optimum Nutrition Bible"*, Patrick Holford, Piatkus, 1997

- *"Balancing Hormones Naturally"*, Kate Neil & Patrick Holford, Piatkus, 1998

- *"Solved: The Riddle of Illness (Your Amazing Thyroid)"*, Stephen E. Langer MD, Keats, 1995

- *"The Bitter Pill"*, Dr. Ellen Grant, Corgi, 1986

- *"The Healing Sun"*, Richard Hobday, Findhorn, 1999

- *"The Silent Passage: Menopause"*, Gail Sheehy, Harper Collins, 1994

- *"Natural Woman, Natural Menopause"*, Marcus Laux ND & Christine Conrad, Pocket Books, 1999

- *"Living Magically"*, *"Stepping into the Magic"* and *"Pure Bliss"*, Gill Edwards, Piatkus, 1991, 1993, 1999

- *"The Creation of Health"* and *"Why People don't Heal, and How they can"*, Caroline Myss, Ph.D. Bantam books, 1999 and 1997

REFERENCES

1. Colborn, T., D. Dumanoski, J.P. Myers. 1996. Hormonal Sabotage. Also published in Natural History, March 1996, 105(3):42-49
2. Estrogens in Unexpected Places: Possible Implications for Researchers and Consumers presented at the Symposium on Estrogens in the Environment, III: Global Health Implications held 9-11 January 1994 in Washington, DC. Also Environ Health Perspect 103(Suppl 7):129-133(1995).
3. F.H. Comhaire, W. Dhooge, A. Mahmoud, C.Depuydt: Een strategie voor de preventie van mannelijke infertiliteit. Verhandelingen van de Koninklijke Academie voor Geneeskunde van België, 1999;LXI:441-455
4. Environment News Service, 30 July 2001, Environment Data Services Ltd, London.
5. Environment News Service, 20 September 2000, Environment Data Services Ltd, London.
6. Office for National Statistics, Mortality Statistics: Cause. England and Wales 1996(1997)
7. American Cancer Society Breast Cancer Facts & Figures
8. I.Gerhard und B.Runnebaum. Grenzen der Hormonsubstitution bei Schadstoffbelastung und Fertilitatsstorungen. Zentralblatt fur Gynakologie, Vol. 114(1992):593-602
9. Theo Colborn and others. Developmental Effects of Endocrine-disrupting Chemicals in Wildlife and Humans. Environmental Health Perspectives, Vol. 101, No. 5 (October 1993):378-384
10. Lee, J.R., MD, The Theory of Estrogen Dominance. Seminar given at St. Thomas's Hospital, London, June 4 1994.
11. IFST: Institute of Food Science & Technology (UK): Phytoestrogens: Information Statement dated October 2001
12. Barbour Warren, Ph.D, Research Associate, Program on Breast Cancer and Environmental Risk Factors, Cornell University (1989-99)
13. Ingram D., Sander, K., Kolybaba, M., and Lpez, D. (1997). Case-control study of phytoestrogens and breast cancer. Lancet 350, 990-994.
14. Arthur J. Vander, James H. Sherman, Dorothy S. Luciano. Human Physiology: The mechanisms of body function. Fourth Edition, McGraw-Hill International Editions, Biological Sciences Series, 1986.
15. Forsling, Akerlund and Stromberg. Variations in plasma concentrations of vasopressin during the menstrual cycle. Journal of Endocrinology 89:263-266 (1981).
16. Marcus Laux, ND & Christine Conrad. Natural woman, Natural menopause. Pocket Books, 1997.
17. Autoimmunity and Women's Health: Is the Female Immune System Different? An interview with Robert G. Lahita, Md, PhD. Women's Health in Primary Care, Vol 4, No. 2/February 2001
18. Peter Parish. Medical Treatments: the benefits and risks. The complete reference guide to drug treatments. Penguin Books, 1991, page 891
19. Alvin H. Folingstad, MD. Estriol, the forgotten estrogen? JAMA, January 1978. 239, 1:29-30
20. Kate Neil & Patrick Holford. Balancing hormones naturally. Piatkus 1998

21. Lemon, H.M., et al. 1966. Reduced estriol excretion in patients with breast cancer prior to endocrine therapy. JAMA 196:1128-1136

22. Lemon, H.M. 1980. Pathophysiologic considerations in the treatment of menopausal patients with oestrogens ; the role of oestriol in the prevention of mammary carcinoma. Act Etidocrinol Suppl 233:17-27

23. Klopper, A. 1980. The risk of endometrial carcinoma from oestrogen therapy of the menopause. Acta Endicrinol Supp 233:29-35

24. London, R.S., et al. 1981. Endocrine parameters and alpha-tocopherol therapy of patients with mammary dysplasia. Cancer Res 41:3811-2813

25. Alp,C.1982. Dietary vitamin E intake and mammary carcinogenesis in rats. Carcinogenesis 3:1453-1456.

26. Weir RJ Jr, Fisher RS. Toxicological studies on borax and boric acid. Toxicol Appl Pharmacol 1972;23:351-64

27. John R. Lee M.D., Medical Letter February 2000. Study shows breast cancer risk for women using HRT. www.JohnLeeMD.com

28. Physician's Desk Reference. 1995. Side effects of Provera (medroxyprogesterone acetate). Taken from Passage to Power. Leslie Kenton. Vermilion 1996

29. What Doctors Don't Tell You. Volume 4, No. 10. HRT More Bad News. Lynne McTaggart.

30. WHI, Women's Health Initiative Investigators. Risks and Benefits of Estrogen Plus Progestin in Healthy Postmenopausal Women. JAMA. 2002;288:321-333

31. Natural Alternatives to HRT. Marilyn Glenville. Greenwhich Editions. 1998.

32. John R. Lee M.D., Medical Letter February 2000. Yet another spin on the conventional medicine point of view. Six errors underlying the conventional HRT paradigm. www.JohnLeeMD.com

33. John R. Lee M.D., Jesse Hanley, M.D., and Virginia Hopkins. PMS and progesterone. Excerpted from What Doctors may not tell you about PREmenopause: Balance your hormones and your life from thirty to fifty. Warner Books. 1999. www.JohnLeeMD.com

34. John R. Lee M.D., Medical Letter 2000. Special report. Saliva vs. serum plasma testing for progesterone

35. John R. Lee M.D., Medical Letter 2000. Progesterone Pulsing and Saliva Hormone Testing. Timing is everything.

36. Elias F. Ilyia, Ph.D., Deborah McLure, C.Sc., and Michel Y. Farhat, Ph.D. Diagnos-Techs Inc. Copyright 2000. Long-term Effects of Topical Progesterone Cream Application. A Case Study.

37. Jeffrey S. Bland, Ph.D. Seminar: Nutritional Improvement of Health Outcomes. The Inflammatory Disorders. 1997. HealthComm, Inc.

38. Doll H; Brown S; Thurston A; Vessey M. Pyridoxine (vitamin B6) and the premenstrual syndrome: a randomized crossover trial. J R Coll Gen Pract, 1989 Sep, 39:326, 364-8

39. Facchinetti F; Borella P; Sances G; Fioroni L; Nappi RE; Genazzani AR Oral magnesium successfully relieves premenstrual mood changes. Obstet Gynecol, 1991 Aug, 78:2, 177-81

40. Muneyvirci Delale O; Nacharaju VL; Altura BM; Altura BT. Sex steroid hormones modulate serum ionized magnesium and calcium levels throughout the menstrual cycle in women. Fertil Steril, 1998 May, 69:5, 958-62

41. Thys-Jacobs S, Starkey P, Bernstein D, Tian J. Calcium carbonate and the premenstrual syndrome: effects on premenstrual and menstrual symptoms. Am J Obstet Gynecol 1998 Aug;179(2):444-52

42. London RS; Sundaram GS; Murphy L; Goldstein PJ The effect of alpha-tocopherol on premenstrual symptomatology: a double-blind study. J Am Coll Nutr, 1983, 2:2, 115-22

43. Chuong CJ; Dawson EB. Zinc and copper levels in premenstrual syndrome. Fertil Steril, 1994 Aug, 62:2, 313-20

44. Harel, Z.; Biro, F., et al.supplementation with omega-3 polyunsaturated fatty acids in the management of dysmenorrhea in adolescents. Am J Ob Gyn 1996;174:1335-1338

45. Dr. Ellen Grant. The Bitter Pill. How Safe is the 'Perfect Contraceptive'? Corgi Books. 1985

46. BBC News Report: Health. 23 March 2002. Pill increases breast cancer risk. http://news.bbc.co.uk/1/hi/health/1887665.stm

47. Leon Chaitow, N.D., D.O., M.B.N.O.A. Candida Albicans. Could Yeast be your Problem? Thorson, 1985

48. Dr Zoltan P Rona MD, MSc . Altered Immunity & The Leaky Gut Syndrome www.health-n-energy.com

49. Leo Galland M.D., F.A.C.N., Director, Foundation for Integrated Medicine. Leaky Gut Syndromes: Breaking the Vicious Cycle (Author of Power Healing: Use The New Integrated Medicine to Heal Yourself, Random House, 1997)

50. National Candida Society. Founded by Dr. Christine Tomlinson, an ex-sufferer, PO Box 151, Orpington, Kent BR5 1UJ, United Kingdom. +44 (0) 1689-813039, e-mail: info@candida-society.org.uk, website: www.candida-society.org.uk

51. Endocronologist, Dr. Phyllis Saifer, M.D., mentioned in "Abstracts from the 16th Annual International Symposium on Man and His Environment in Health and Disease – 1998". http://www.aehf.com/articles/98sympabs.htm

52. Kristi NewMyer, MD. Endometriosis. http://altmed.creighton.edu/endometriosis/about_endometriosis.htm

53. Current Approaches to Endometriosis, Patient Care, Jan. 15, 1997, pp.34-38

54. National Kidney and Urologic Diseases Information Clearinghouse website: http://www.niddk.nih.gov/health/urolog/pubs/cystitis/cystitis.htm

55. Dr. Jonathan Brostoff and Linda Gamlin. The complete guide to Food Allergy and Intolerance. Bloomsbury Publishing. 1989.

56. Leon Chaitow, N.D., D.O., M.B.N.O.A.. Stone Age Diet. The Natural Way to Eat. Macdonald Optima. 1987

57. Broda O. Barnes, M.D., and Lawrence Galton. Hypothyroidism: the unsuspected illness. Harper and Row. 1976

58. Karen Goodfellow, BSc, Bed(Hons) DPSN. Research Officer for Thyroid UK and Senior Lecturer at the University of Northumbria in Newscastle. Underactive thyroid. A nutritional approach. Optimum Nutrition Journal Vol. 15, No. 2, Summer 2002, pages 24-30.

59. Dr. John Lowe. The Metabolic Treatment of Fibromyalgia. McDowell Publishing.

60. Stephen E. Langer, M.D., and James F. Scheer. Solved: The riddle of illness. Your amazing thyroid and how you can work with it to control arthritis, obesity, depression, diabetes, heart disease and circulatory problems, cancer, sexual problems. Keats Publishing 2000.

61. Daniel R. Doerge, Ph.D., a researcher at the Food and Drug Aministration's National Center for Toxicological Research. Natural Health magazine. March 1999

62. Divi RL; Chang HC; Doerge DR. Anti-thyroid isoflavones from soybean: isolation, characterization, and mechanisms of action. National Center for Toxicological Research, Jefferson, AR 72079, USA, Biochem Pharmacol, 1997 Nov, 54:10, 1087-96)

63. Forsythe WA. Soy Protein, thyroid regulation and cholesterol metabolism. Forsythe WA. Soy protein, thyroid regulation and cholesterol metabolism. J Nutr 1995;125:619S–23S.

64. Bennink MR, Mayle JE, Bourquin LD, Thiagarajan D. Evaluation of soy protein in risk reduction for colon cancer and cardiovascular disease: Preliminary results. Second International Symposium on the Role of Soy in Preventing and Treating Chronic Disease. September 15–18, 1996. Brussels, Belgium

65. Mary Shomon. www.thyroid-info.com

66. Zoeller R.R. Polychlorinated biphenyls as disruptors of thyroid hormone action. Department of Biology and Molecular Cellular Biology Program, University of Massachusetts, Amherts, Massachusetts.
www.bio.umass.edu/biology.zoeller/pcbreveiw/htm

67. Thyroid UK. www.thyroiduk.org

68. A.G. Awad, MD, BCH, PhD, FRCP(C) Associate Professor of Psychiatry, University of Toronto Director. The Thyroid and the Mind and Emotions/Thyroid Dysfunction and Mental Disorders. Psychobiological Medicine Unit, Department of Psychiatry, Toronto Western Hospital. Summary of an address to the Kitchener-Waterloo Area Chapter

69. Dr. Gordon Skinner. (J Nutr Environ Med, 2000; 10: 115-24). His thyroid treatment is publicised in Tears Behind Closed Doors. Diana Holmes. Avon Books 1998.

70. Dr. Barry Durrant-Peatfield. (J Nutr Environ Med, 1996; 6: 371-8) and his own information booklet: Diagnosis and Treatment of ME.

71. Doris Jones. Thyroid Problems. The link with 21st century deiseases. What Doctors Don't Tell You. Vol 12. No. 9. December 2001. pages 1-4.

72. Marilyn Glenville. Natural alternatives to HRT. Greenwhich Editions. 1997.

73. Leslie Kenton. Passage to Power. Vermilion. 1996.

74. HRT: the myths exploded. HRT: more bad news. What Doctors Don't Tell You. Vol 4. Nos. 9 & 10. Editor/author Lynne McTaggart.

75. Risks and Benefits of Estrogen Plus Progestin in Healthy Postmenopausal Women. Principal Results from the Women's Health Initiative Randomized Controlled Trial. JAMA. July 17, 2002. Vol. 288 No. 3:321-333.

76. Marcus Laux, N.D. and Christine Conrad. Natural Woman, Natural Menopause. Harper Collins. 1997

77. Jonathan Wright M.D. and John Morgenthaler. Don't let your doctor give you horse urine! There are better treatments for menopause.
http://smart-drugs.net/ias-esnatri.htm

78. Vander ArthurJ. Human Physiology, The Mechanisms of Body Function. Fourth Edition. McGraw-Hill International. 1998.

79. Henry Osiecki. The Physicians Handbook of Clinical Nutrition. Bio Concepts. 1990

80. National Osteoporosis Society. Camerton, Bath, BA2 0PJ. www.nos.org.uk

81. Susan Ott, MD, Associate Professor Department of Medicine University of Washington. Bone Mineral Density. BMJ. April 9, 1994

82. John R Lee, MD and Virginia Hopkins. The truth about Osteoporosis.
www.johnleemd.com/trutabos.htm

83. British National Formulary. BNF 43 March 2002. www.bnf.org
84. Cummings SR, Nevitt MC, Browner WS, Stone K, Fox KM. Ensrud KE, Cauley J, Black D, and Vogt TM for the Study of Osteoporotic Fractures Research Group. Risk Factors for Hip Fracture in White Women. N Engl J Med 1995; 332:767-73
85. Richard A. Passwater, PhD, and Elmer M. Cranton, M.D. Trace Elements, Hair Analysis and Nutrition. Keats Publishing. 1983.
86. Ettinger B, Pak CY, Citron JT, et al. Potassium-magnesium citrate is an effective prophylaxis against recurrent calcium oxalate nephrolithiasis. J Urol. 1997;158:2069-2073
87. HJ, Greer LG, Haynes SD, et al. Pharmacokinetic and Pharmacodynamic Comparison of Two Calcium Supplements in Postmenopausal Women. Heller JclinPharmacol. 2000; 40:1237-1244
88. Cur Res in Osteo and Bone Mine Meas II, British Institute Radiology, London, 1992
89. Burnell JM, Baylink DJ, Chesnut CH III, Teubner EJ. The role of skeletal calcium deficiency in post menopausal osteoporosis. Calcif Tissue Int 1986; 38:187-92
90. Hosking DJ, Ross PD, Thompson DE, et al. Evidence that increased calcium intake does not prevent early postmenopausal bone loss. Clin Ther 1998;20:933-44
91. Abraham GE, Grewal H. A total dietary program emphasizing magnesium instead of calcium. J Reprod Med 1990;35:503–7.Recker RR. Calcium absorption and achlorhydria. N Engl J Med 1985; 313(2):70-3.
92. PCRM. The Physicians Committee for Responsible Medicine. www.pcrm.org
93. Feskanich D, Willett WC, Stampfer MJ, Colditz GA. Milk, dietary calcium, and bone fractures in women: a 12-year prospective study. Am J Publ Health 1997;87:992-7
94. Cumming RG, Klineberg RJ. Case-control study of risk factors for hip fractures in the elderly. Am J Epidemiol 1994;139:493-505
95. Weinster RL, and Krumdieck CL. Dairy foods and bone health: examination of the evidence. American Journal of Clinical Nutrition. 2000;72:681-9.
96. Cramer DW, Willett WC, Bell DA, et al. Galactose consumption and metabolism in relation to the risk of ovarian cancer. Lancet 1989;2:66-71.
97. Simoons FJ. A geographic approach to senile cataracts: possible links with milk consumption, lactase activity, and galactose metabolism. Digestive Diseases and Sciences 1982;27:257-64
98. Couet C, Jan P, Debry G. Lactose and cataract in humans: a review. J Am Coll Nutr 1991;10:79-86.
99. Kate Neil and Patrick Holford. Balancing Hormones Naturally. Piatkus. 1998
100. The UK Vegetarian Society. Parkdale, Dunham Road, Altrincham, Cheshire, WA14 4QG. www.vegsoc.org
101. Virginia Worthington, M.S., Sc.D., C.N.S. Nutritional Quality of Organic Versus Conventional Fruits, Vegetables, and Grains. The Jouranl of Alternative and Complementary Medicine. Volume 7, Number 2, 2001, pp. 161–173
102. UK Soil Association. www.soilassociation.org
103. Zarkadas M, Geougeon-Reyburn R, Marliss EB, et al. Sodium chloride supplementation and urinary calcium excretion in post menopausal women. Am J Clin Nutr 1989;50:1088-94
104. Wyshak G, Frisch RE. Carbonated beverages, dietary calcium, the dietary calcium/phosphorous ratio, and bone fractures in girls and boys. J Adolescent Health 1994;15:210-5

105. Mazariegos-Ramos E, Guerrero-Romero F, Rodriquez-Moran F, et al. Consumption of soft drinks with phosphoric acid as a risk factor for the development of hypocalcaemia in children: a case-control study. J Pediatr 1995;126:940-2

106. Shuster J, Jenkins A, Logan C, et al. Soft drink consumption and urinary stone recurrence: a randomized prevention trial. J Clin Epidemiol 1992;45:911-6

107. Hernandez-Avila M, Colditz GA, Stampfer MJ, et al. Caffeine, moderate alcohol intake, and risk of the hip and forearm in middle-aged women. Am J Clin Nutri1991;54:157-63

108. Kynast-Gales SA, Massey LK. Effect of caffeine on circadian excretion of urinary calcium and magnesium. J Am CollNutr 1994;13:467-72

109. Harris SS, Dawson-Hughes B. Caffeine and bone loss in healthy postmenopausal women. Am J Clin Nutr 1994;60:573-8

110. Feskanich D, Willett WC, Stampfer MJ, Coldtiz GA. Protein consumption and bone fractures in women. Am J Epidemiol1996;143:472-9

111. Schurch M-A, Rizzoli R, Slosman D, et al. Protein supplements increase serum insulin-like growth factor-I levels and attenuate proximal femur bone loss in patients with recent hip fracture. A randomised double blind placebo controlled trial.Ann Intern Med1998;128:801-9)

112. Phillip Day. Cancer. Why we're still dying to know the truth. Credence Publications. 2001

113. Dr. John Yiamouyiannis. Fluoride, The Aging Factor. Health Action Press. 1993

114. Gaby Alan R. MD and Wright Jonathan V. MD. Nutrients and osteoporosis. Review Article. Journal of Nutritional Medicine 1990;1:63-72

115. Richard Hobday. The Healing Sun. Findhorn Press. 1999

116. Weir RJ Jr, Fisher RS. Toxicologic studies on borax and boric acid. Toxicol Appl Pharmacol 1972;23:351-64

117. Chow R, Harrison JE, Noorarius C. Effect of two randomised exercise programmes on bone mass of healthy post menopausal women Br Med J 1987;295:1441-4

118. Lee, John R. MD. Osteoporosis reversal: the role of progesterone. Int Clin Nutr Rev 1990;10:384-91

119. Prior J C. Progesterone as a bone-trophic hormone. Endocr Rev 1990;11:386-98

120. van Papendorp DH, Coetzer H, Kruger MC. Biochemical profile of osteoporotic patients on essential fatty acid supplementation. Nutr Res 1995;15:325-34

121. Kruger MC, Coetzer H, de Winter R, et al. Calcium, gamma-linolenic acid and eicosapentaenoic acid supplementation in senile osteoporosis. Aging 1998;10:385-94

122. Gennari C, Agnusdei D, Crepaldi G, et al. Effect of ipriflavone – a synthetic derivative of natural isoflavones – on bone mass loss in the early years after menopause. Menopause 1998;5(1):9-15

123. Agnusdei D, Buffalini L. Efficacy of ipriflavone in established osteoporosis and long term safety. Calcif Tissue Int 1997;61 :142-147

124. Alexandersen P, Toussaint A, Christiansen C, et al. Ipriflavone in the treatment of postmenopausal osteoporosis: a randomized controlled trial. JAMA.2001;285:1482-1488

125. World Health Organisation. 1999. Food Safety Issues associated with Products from Aquaculture. WHO Technical Report #883, Geneva

126. U.S. Food and Drug Adminstration Nutrition Database. www.fda.gov

127. Consumer Advisory Center for Food Safety and Applied Nutrition, U.S. An Important Message for Pregnant Women and Women of childbearing age who may become preganant about the Risks of Mercury in Fish. Food and Drug Administration March 2001

128. Dr. Joseph Mercola. No safe level of trans fat. July 2002. www.mercola.com/2002/jul/27/trans_fat.htm

129. Dr. Udo Erasmus. Fats that Heal, Fats that Kill. Alive Books. www.savant-health.com

130. Liz Earle. New Vital Oils. Vermilion. 2002.

131. Mary G. Enig, Ph.D, Director of the Nutritional Sciences Division of Enig Associates, Inc., Silver Spring, Marylan, and President of the Maryland Nutritionists Association. "Health Risks from Processed Foods and the Dangers of Trans Fats. Dr. Mary Enig interviewed by Richard A. Passwater, Ph.D. www.mercola.com/2000/june/10/trans_fats.htm

132. Warburg O. "On the origin of cancer cells." Science 1956 Feb;123:309-14

133. Bland, Jeffrey S. PhD., Nutritional Improvement of Health Outcomes – The Inflammatory Disorders. Chapter 2. HealthComm Seminar Series 1997.

134. Ann de Wees Allen, N.D., Director of Research and Development, The Glycemic Research Institute. The Glycemic Table. 25 June 1998

135. Ray C. Wunderlich Jr., M.D. Sugar and your Health. Good Health Publications. 1982

136. National Transportation Safety Board and NASA Ames Research Center. Fatigue Symposium Proceedings. November 1-2, 1995.

137. Singletary Keith, PhD and Gapstur Susan, PhD. "Alcohol and Breast Cancer". JAMA 286, 17: 2143-2151

138. Feigelson Heather, PhD. "Alcohol Consumption Increases The Risks of Fatal Breast Cancer". Cancer Causes and Control. December 2002. www.cancer.org.

139. Dr. Bernard Jensen March 25, 1908 - February 22, 2001. Bernard Jensen International and Natural Books & Products, 1914 W. Mission Road, Suite F, Escondido, California, 92029, US. www.bernardjensen.org

140. Sara Martin quoting Dr. Bernard Jensen. A Process of Elimination. Here's Health March 1988

141. Bradlow HL, Sepkovic DW, Telang NT, Osborne MP. Multifunctional aspects of the action of indole-3-carbinol as an antitumor agent. Ann N Y Acad Sci 1999;889:204–13.

142. Bradlow HL, Sepkovic DW, Telang NT, Osborne MP. Indole-3-carbinol. A novel approach to breast cancer prevention. Ann N Y Acad Sci 1995;768:180–200.

143. www.gnc.com/health_notes/Supp/Indole_3_Carbinol.htm

144. Eden J, et al. Hormonal effect of isoflavones. Program & Abstract Book, Second International Symposium on the Role of Soy in Preventing and Treating Chronic Disease, Sept 15-18, 1996, Brussels, Belgium: 41-42.

145. Burke GL. The potential use of a dietary soy supplement as a post-menopausal hormone replacement therapy. Program & Abstract Book, Second International Symposium on the Role of Soy in Preventing and Treating Chronic Disease, Sept 15-18, 1996, Brussels, Belgium: 40-41.

146. Honoré EK, et al. Soy isoflavones enhance coronary vascular reactivity in atherosclerotic female macaques. Fertility and Sterility, 1997;67:148-154.

147. Murrill WB, et al. Prepubertal genistein exposure suppresses mammary cancer and enhances gland differentiation in rats. Carcinogenesis, 1996;17:1451-1457.

148. David Hoffmann. Thorsons Guide to Medical Herbalism. Thorsons. 1991
149. Yost, David A., 1989. Clinical Safety of Aspartame. American Family Physician, Volume 39, Number 2, pages 201-206, 1989.
150. U.S. Department of Health and Human Services released the listing adverse reactions reported to the FDA (DHHS 1994).

INDEX

A

absorption 3, 5, 17, 40, 43, 46, 49, 51, 57, 76, 88, 99-102, 105, 112, 114, 118, 131, 134, 151, 194
acid reflux 15, 151
acid-forming foods 9, 96, 98
acidophilus 15, 154
acne 8, 33, 39-40, 66, 114, 156-157
Addison's disease 4, 51
adrenals 1, 19, 23-24, 27, 30-31, 37, 65, 73, 85, 120, 137, 149, 153
alcohol 4, 7, 15, 17, 37, 40-41, 43, 48, 54, 59, 61-63, 79, 81, 86, 88, 91, 96-99, 103, 106-107, 115, 125, 132, 135, 138, 141-145, 195-196
aldosterone 1, 27-28, 31
alkaline phosphatase 9, 90, 92, 102
alkaline-forming foods 9, 97
allergies 3, 8, 14-15, 46, 49-50, 54, 60-62, 67, 75, 77, 119, 123, 127, 136
allergy pulse test 8, 62-64, 70, 93, 112
alpha linolenic acid 5
amalgam fillings 5, 48, 156
amenorrhoea (lack of periods) 1, 14, 136, 145
anal itching 14, 49
androgens 13, 30, 73, 85, 133
anorexia 9, 86, 136
anovulatory periods 21, 32, 72-73
antacids 8, 69
anthocyanidins 10, 13, 143
antibiotics 14, 48, 53, 92, 102, 106, 113-114, 153
anti-candida programme 4, 51-53
anti-convulsants 8, 69
anti-fungal 4, 51, 134, 167
anti-oxidants 10, 111, 120, 156
anxiety 14, 16, 32-33, 39, 54, 75-76, 83, 89, 123, 136, 138, 141, 155
APICH 14, 50-51
appetite 8, 65, 114, 145, 148, 156, 168-169, 175
apricots 9, 94, 117, 169, 173, 175

Armour thyroid 8, 70
arthritis 1, 28, 51, 123, 192
artificial lighting 5, 17, 41, 157
aspartame 4, 58-59, 143, 166, 197
asthma 33, 50, 57, 60, 62, 68, 82, 86, 136, 145
athlete's foot 14, 50
autoimmunity 14, 51, 190
autotoxicity 15, 153
avocados 9, 107, 117-118, 121, 129, 147

B

B vitamins 1, 29, 37, 40, 42, 49, 68, 71, 78, 109, 118, 132, 141-143, 145, 153, 155
back pain 5
bad breath 4, 54, 153
baking 13, 121-122, 128, 166
barley 9, 22, 62, 111-112
Barnes basal temperature test 8, 70
beta blockers 8, 69
betaine hydrochloride 4, 15, 51, 100-101, 106, 151-152
bilberry extract 13, 143
bile 15, 35, 101, 152
bioflavinoids 158, 174
bisphosphonates 9, 87
black cohosh 15, 161-162
bloating 1, 16, 32-33, 39-40, 49, 52, 54, 57, 66, 75, 112, 148, 151
blood sugar 3, 5, 40-42, 46, 50, 53, 57, 61, 67, 77-78, 82, 113, 115, 117-118, 123, 130-142, 145, 147-150, 155-156, 169
body odour 4, 54
bone protection plan 9, 106
borlotti beans 9, 113, 173, 176-177, 183
boron 4, 30, 84, 91, 101, 103, 106, 156, 158
bowel tolerance 15, 154
brain chemistry 5, 42, 132, 145
breast cancer 4, 13, 19, 21-22, 28-30, 32-34, 37, 43, 45-47, 74, 79-80, 82, 88, 92, 119, 127, 131, 143-144, 160-161, 189-192, 196
breast tenderness 5, 33, 39-40, 43, 83, 144, 146, 156, 158
breathing 5, 41, 47

breathlessness 15, 156
buckwheat 9, 62, 96, 111-112, 166, 173
butter 15, 20, 93, 95-96, 107, 115, 121-122, 127-128, 131, 135, 146, 165-166, 173

C

caffeine 5, 15, 37, 40-41, 43, 81, 86, 88, 97-100, 115, 120, 131-132, 135, 138, 141-142, 146, 148, 169, 195
calcitonin 9, 84, 87, 105
calcitrol 9, 87
calcium 4, 28, 33, 37, 40, 42-43, 78, 81, 83-107, 110, 112, 115, 117-120, 145, 150-151, 154-156, 158, 166, 191-192, 194-195
calcium carbonate 9, 89-90, 98, 107, 192
calcium citrate 9, 90, 107, 158
calcium citrate malate 9, 90
calcium oxalate crystals 9, 90
candida 3, 5, 48-53, 55-59, 62, 133, 192
candidiasis checklist 4, 53
carbohydrates 5, 46, 49, 59, 75, 106, 111-112, 116, 119, 129, 131, 134, 139, 149, 151-152, 164
cardiovascular disease 8, 28, 80-81, 88, 127, 193
cervical cancer 4, 7, 13-14, 161
cheese 15-17, 20, 62-63, 92-93, 95-96, 115, 121-122, 148-149, 163-164, 168, 170
chick peas 9, 94, 113, 173, 176, 185
chocolate 4-5, 16-17, 37, 41, 59, 62, 91, 96-100, 106-107, 114, 117, 129-130, 132-135, 140-142, 146-148, 153, 164
cholesterol 4-5, 27-28, 31, 33, 37, 65, 67, 69, 81, 83, 115, 117, 125, 128, 152-153, 193
choline 4, 29, 126
chromium 4, 13, 42, 115, 118, 132, 134, 141-142, 150, 155, 158
chronic fatigue 5, 14, 50, 57, 66
cis fatty acids 5, 126, 128
cocoa 5, 37, 99-100, 122, 132, 141, 146
coffee 5, 7, 16-17, 59, 61-63, 78-79, 91, 96, 98, 106-107, 115, 120, 125, 132-133,

135, 140-142, 145-148, 167
cold pressed oils 5, 43, 75, 107, 126-129, 165, 170, 186
collagen 4, 28, 84, 103
colon 15, 29, 152-155, 193
colon cleanse 15, 153-154
colonic irrigation 15, 154
concentrated carbohydrates 9, 111-112
concentration 8, 14, 27, 35, 39, 60, 75, 115, 123, 138, 147
conjugated linoleic acid (CLA) 13, 127
conjugated oestrogens 4, 30
constipation 4, 16, 49, 51-52, 54, 57, 66, 87, 118, 152, 154
convenience foods 9, 111, 163
copper 5, 9, 43, 84, 91, 103, 192
corn (maize) 9, 75, 111-112, 124, 127, 152, 166, 168, 173, 176-177, 180-181
corticosterone 4, 19, 27-28, 31
cortisol 4, 27-28, 31, 37, 41, 85, 137
cottage cheese 9, 62, 93, 95, 168, 170
coumestan 4, 22
cramping 5, 14, 40, 43, 71, 116, 145, 154-155
cravings 1, 16, 39-41, 51, 54, 110, 117, 130, 135, 142-143, 147, 150, 156, 166
cruciferous vegetables 15, 161
cystitis 4, 50, 53, 58-59, 83, 192
cysts 4, 13-14, 29, 33, 50, 133, 161

D

dairy produce 5, 17, 40, 61, 91, 93, 106, 110, 119, 128, 133, 153, 164, 166
depression 4, 13-14, 32-33, 36, 39-40, 42-43, 45, 50-51, 54, 58, 60, 67, 76, 83, 114, 123, 136, 138, 141, 146, 155, 192
detoxification 15, 35, 102, 115, 149, 152-153, 162
dextrose 9, 113, 143, 166
DHEA 27-28, 30-31, 37-38, 133-134
diabetes 5, 42, 67, 76, 82, 123, 131, 133, 142, 192
diarrhoea 14, 49, 54, 58-59, 71, 87
diazepam 8, 69
Didronel 87
digestion 3, 5, 17, 40, 46, 49, 51, 57, 76, 151

L

lactose 13, 92, 143, 154, 194
leaky gut 8, 14-15, 40, 49-51, 53, 61-63, 77, 123, 192
lecithin 15, 115, 126
lectins 9, 112
Levodopa 8, 69
Levothyroxine 8, 70
l-glutamine 4, 51, 71, 145, 150
l-glycine 8, 71
LH 4, 25-26, 73-74
libido (sex drive) 8, 32, 73, 76
lignans 6, 22, 118
Lindane 9, 92
linoleic acid 8, 124, 127
linseed 7, 22, 75, 79, 97, 105, 122, 125, 128, 147, 160, 186
linseed oil 15, 79, 105, 128, 160, 186
Liothyronine 70
liquorice 8, 38, 160, 162
lithium 4, 69
liver 6, 28-29, 33, 35, 42, 65-66, 73, 82, 86, 102, 115, 131, 135, 141-143, 145, 153, 155, 158, 162
loss of appetite 15, 65, 114, 156
low blood pressure 4, 51, 67, 138
low blood sugar 7, 40-41, 77, 118, 132, 138-139, 149-150
low stomach acid 8, 40, 86, 88, 100, 151
low thyroid function 3, 8, 21, 32, 46, 50-51, 65, 68-70, 77, 120, 135, 156
l-tyrosine 4, 51, 71
Lupus 7, 28

M

magnesium 8, 37, 40, 42-43, 78, 84, 89-93, 96-97, 100-102, 106-107, 115-116, 118-119, 126, 134, 136, 141-143, 145-146, 150, 154-155, 158, 191, 194-195
malabsorption 86
manganese 7, 9, 42, 84, 91, 103, 132, 141-142, 150, 155-156, 158
margarine 15, 20, 105, 121-122, 127-128
medroxyprogesterone 8, 32, 80, 191
memory 8, 14, 54, 60, 67, 75, 115, 123, 138

menopause 3, 7-8, 13-14, 25, 30-32, 34, 37, 48, 72-82, 85-86, 89, 132, 138, 141, 144, 160-162, 188-191, 193, 195
menorrhagia 14
menstrual cycle 7, 21, 23-25, 31-32, 43, 190-191
menstruation 13, 26, 58, 67, 72, 188
mental stability 3, 7, 12-13, 77, 136, 141
mercury 4, 8, 48, 69, 114, 156-157, 196
methyl mercury 9, 114
methylparabens 13, 129
migraines 14, 39, 54, 66, 129
milk 8, 20, 33, 62-64, 68, 90-96, 99, 115, 119, 127-128, 154, 162, 167-169, 173, 180-181, 194
milk thistle (silymarin) 15, 162
millet 4, 62, 68, 96-97, 111-112, 148, 166, 168, 173
mineral oil 13, 110, 129
miscarriage 15, 67, 123
miso 4, 22, 62, 68, 119, 176
molasses 9, 114
monounsaturated fat 15, 122
mood swings 8, 14, 32, 39-40, 42-43, 45, 54, 60, 72, 76, 138, 146
muscle pain 8, 75

N

nails 4, 40, 50, 53, 57, 66, 114-115, 123, 128, 151, 156
natural progesterone 8, 19, 34-37, 56-57, 82, 104, 134, 160, 162
nausea 15
nervous system 9, 65, 84, 110, 116, 120, 141, 144, 166
neurotransmitters 8, 42
night blindness 4, 67
night sweats 8, 14, 32, 72, 75, 77-79, 131, 138, 160, 162
nightshade family 8, 62-63, 135
nitrites 9, 113
norri flakes 9, 15, 120, 176, 178, 182, 187
nutritional deficiencies 3, 8, 15, 17, 21, 40, 42, 46, 73, 77, 87-88, 155
nutritional stressors 8, 13, 17, 40, 59, 73, 141, 146, 149, 155-156, 164

nuts 8, 21-22, 43, 62, 75, 78, 94-97, 100, 107, 110-112, 116, 118-119, 121-122, 125, 128-131, 133, 135, 147-149, 153, 165-168, 173, 175, 177, 181

O

oats 9, 22, 62, 96, 111-112, 135, 149, 153, 167-168, 173
oestradiol (E2) 8, 27-30, 74, 81-82, 143, 152
oestriol (E3) 8, 27-30, 43, 82, 103, 118, 155, 191
oestrogen 8-9, 18-23, 25-31, 33-34, 37, 41-43, 45, 50, 56-58, 69-70, 72-82, 84-88, 91, 103, 105, 119, 133, 138, 143, 156, 160-162, 191
oestrogen dominance 8, 18-21, 31, 34, 57, 74, 77, 160
oestrogen mimics 8, 18, 20
oestrone (E1) 8, 28-29, 81-82
oil refining 13, 105, 126
olive oil 15, 107, 121-122, 126-129, 165-166, 171, 173, 176-186
omega-3 fatty acids 8, 37, 81, 114, 118, 125, 159-160
omega-6 fatty acids 124
optimum nutrition 2-3, 5, 8-9, 11, 36, 46, 65, 71, 97, 108-109, 145, 152, 188-189, 192
oral contraceptives (the Pill) 8, 46
organic 9, 20, 75, 93, 106, 114-115, 127, 129, 155, 160, 164-165, 168, 173-174, 194
osteoblasts 9, 84-85, 105
osteoclasts 9, 84, 105
osteoporosis 3, 8, 13-14, 19, 21, 30, 32, 34, 36, 79, 81, 84-92, 97-101, 104-106, PB 154, 156, 160, 194-196
ovaries 1, 13-14, 19, 23-25, 27-28, 30-31, 65, 72-73, 79, 82, 86, 92, 133, 156
oxalic acid 9, 99-100
oxidation 9, 118

P

pallor 4, 66, 138
palpitations 4, 67, 71, 138
pancreas 14, 49, 131, 133, 142

panic attacks 8, 32, 39, 76
paraffinium 13, 129
parathyroid hormone 9, 84-85, 87
Parkinson's disease 4, 69, 166
pau d'arco 4, 59
PCBs 8, 19-20, 55, 69
peanuts 9, 62, 96, 111-112, 119
peri-menopause 4, 72, 79
period pains (dysmenorrhoea) 15, 56, 129, 155, 160
periods 8-9, 13-14, 16, 39-41, 45-46, 51, 67, 70, 72-73, 79, 133-134, 136, 145, 156, 158, 160-161
pesticides 8, 15, 18, 20, 41, 92-93, 115
petrochemical derivatives 13, 18, 41, 129
petrolatum 13, 129
phosphorous 9, 98, 105, 195
Photon Absorptionmetry 9, 86
phytic acid 9, 99-100, 112
phytoestrogens 8, 15, 21-22, 31, 119, 160-161, 190
phytohormones 94, 111, 115, 118, 120, 160, 187
Pituitary 8, 23-26, 51, 65, 79, 161
PMS (premenstrual syndrome) 1, 9-10, 13-14, 16, 21, 29, 34, 39-44, 46-47, 50-52, 61, 77, 123-124, 129, 131-132, 138, 141, 143-144, 156, 161, 191
polycystic ovaries 8, 13-14, 133
polyunsaturated fat 15, 122
post-menopause 4, 73
post-menopause zest 8
power foods 9, 110, 117
power naps 13, 140
prednisolone 4, 53, 58
pregnancy 8, 14, 26, 28, 31, 33, 48, 72, 81, 83
pregnenolone 8, 27-28, 31, 37
Premarin 4, 58-59, 80-82
premature ageing 9, 99, 120, 123
probiotics 4, 51
processed foods 42, 61, 91-92, 105, 110, 125, 196
progesterone 8, 10, 19-21, 23-28, 30-37, 41-43, 50-51, 56-57, 72-79, 82, 104, 133-134, 137-138, 160-162, 191, 195
prostoglandins 15
protein 10, 46, 49, 60, 65, 84, 88, 91, 98,

supplements 3, 6, 10, 15, 30, 34, 36-38, 40, 44, 57, 59, 62, 67-68, 71, 76, 78, 88-91, 100-101, 103-104, 106-107, 109, 134, 136, 142-143, 145, 150, 154-155, 157-160, 194-195
sweating 13, 71, 138
synthetic hormones 10, 14, 20, 23, 34, 45, 56, 70

T

T3 8, 65, 69-70
T4 8, 65, 69-70
tamari 4, 62, 68
tea 10, 16-17, 59, 61-63, 78-79, 91, 96, 98, 106-107, 115, 120, 132-133, 140-141, 146-148, 169, 173
tempeh 4, 22, 62, 68, 95, 119
testes 8, 65
testosterone 8-9, 19, 27-28, 31, 37, 73, 85, 87, 133
the Pill 8-9, 14, 18, 20, 40, 43-46, 53, 56, 69, 83, 103, 145, 162
thirst 13, 24, 39, 123, 138
thrush 14, 49-50, 53, 55, 57-59, 133-134
thyroid 3, 8, 21, 23-24, 32, 46, 50-51, 65, 67-71, 77, 81, 84, 86, 110, 120, 130, 135, 156, 189, 192-193
tingling sensation in arms and legs 15, 123
tinnitus 67
tofu 4, 22, 62, 68, 79, 95-96, 119, 128, 135, 149, 161, 170-171, 173-174, 177, 181, 187
tranquilisers 4, 69
trans fatty acids 10, 43, 75, 104-105, 121-122, 126-128, 130
transit time 15, 152
Tri-Est 4, 82
TSH 8, 65, 69

U

unsaturated fat 15, 122
uric acid 9, 90
urticaria 4, 60
uterine cancer 8, 13, 19

V

vaginal discharge 9, 53, 60, 93
vaginal dryness 14-15, 160
vegetables 10, 15, 17-18, 20-22, 42, 46, 68, 75, 78, 93-94, 96-99, 102, 106, 110-112, 114, 116-117, 125, 131, 133, 148-149, 153, 161, 164, 169-170, 173-174, 176-178, 181, 183-184, 186, 194
vegetarians 8, 20, 113-114, 164, 174
vitamin A 4, 68, 158
vitamin B3 10, 42, 126, 141, 155
vitamin B6 10, 42, 83-84, 100-103, 107, 117, 126, 141, 151, 155-156, 191
vitamin C 10, 37, 81, 91, 93, 141, 145, 150, 154, 156, 158
vitamin D 9, 84-85, 87, 91, 101-102, 106, 118, 155, 158
vitamin E 8, 30, 43, 78, 107, 109, 118, 126, 134, 157-158, 191
vitamin K 9, 15, 102, 106, 153
Vitex Agnus Castus 8-9, 136, 161-162

W

water 10, 15, 18, 20, 32, 39-41, 60, 65, 68, 75, 97-99, 103, 106-107, 110, 114-117, 120, 130, 141, 146-147, 151, 154-155, 163, 167-169, 173-174, 176-183
water retention 4, 32, 39, 60, 65, 75, 155
weight gain 8, 13, 16, 21, 32, 39-40, 45, 65, 72, 75, 83, 127, 129-130, 135
weight loss 13, 15, 65, 135
wheat 10, 17, 22, 62-63, 93, 96, 111-112, 134-136, 153, 160, 164-166
wheat intolerance 9, 112
wholefood 9, 106, 109, 142, 154-155
wholegrains 9, 21, 111, 153
wild yam 10, 22, 34, 161-162
World Health Organisation 9, 19, 85, 89, 114, 196

X

xenoestrogens 8, 18-20, 41

Y

yeast infection 4, 10, 48, 53, 55
yoghurt 9, 62, 93, 95, 106, 115, 147, 149,
  154, 168

Z

zinc 10, 37, 40, 42-43, 68-69, 71, 78, 84,
  91, 100-101, 103, 106, 112, 114, 117-
  118, 126, 132, 136, 141-143, 145, 150-
  151, 156, 158, 192